THE STORY
OF A
CANCER CURE

BOOK ONE

By

Thomas Burke Caulfield

The Center For Advanced
Psychic Research and Development, Inc.
Riverhead, New York

Copyright © 1983 by Thomas Burke Caulfield

Library of Congress Cataloging in Publication Data

Caulfield, Thomas Burke, 1943-
　　The story of a cancer cure, book one.

　　1. Mental healing. 2. Cancer--Treatment. I. Title.
RC271.M4C38　　1983　　　616.99'406　　　83-26160
ISBN 0-9611788-0-9

For Information and Ordering, Contact:

　　The Center For Advanced
　　Psychic Research and Development, Inc.
　　P.O. Box 1268
　　Riverhead, New York 11901

Manufactured in the United States of America

ACKNOWLEDGEMENTS

I would like to express my gratitude to friends and to all the members of the Caulfield family for their help, support, and understanding.

TABLE OF CONTENTS

Chapter

THE STORY
OF A
CANCER CURE

BOOK ONE

Chapter One
AN AFFAIR OF LOVE

It is difficult to assign any particular point in time in which a person may choose to become aware or develop his own intuitive abilities and potential. My own active pursuit of intuitive abilities resulted from a series of traumatic events that made me wonder about my life. I would like to present those circumstances as the start of my story of a cancer cure.

In 1967, I was assigned by the U.S. Department of the Army to the United States Army Reception Station at Fort Ord, California. The fort is located on a large tract of land that abuts the Pacific Ocean. Fort Ord, which is south of San Francisco, served as a basic training facility for new army personnel. I was the Quartermaster Supply Officer at the reception station that processed new recruits into the Army.

I was fortunate to live in the nearby town of

Pacific Grove instead of the overcrowded bachelor Officer's Quarters located on the post. The civilian atmosphere was much more appealing to me than life on the army post. Pacific Grove was unique in that no alcoholic beverages could be sold in the town limits. However, just on the outskirts of town were ample liquor stores providing great quantities of booze. No one really seemed to mind the prohibition and the party atmosphere seemed all-pervasive.

There were about sixty apartments that made up the complex in which I lived. I tried to keep up the party tradition by becoming acquainted with all the new female occupants who moved into the complex. I acted as the unofficial "Welcome Wagon" host. After striking up an acquaintance with the girls, I would pop in every week or so for a dinner-time visit. On Wednesdays and Thursdays I visited Diane's. On Friday I was sure to be found at Pat's apartment, and on Saturday or Sunday I would pay Sherri a visit.

One Saturday morning, I noticed a station wagon being unloaded by two new apartment dwellers. I did not get a good look at the first girl, but I knew right away that the skinny, flat-chested, kinky-haired blonde was not my type. Both girls were moving into one of the recently vacated flats in the center of the complex.

I decided to uphold my tradition of welcoming newcomers by making suitable arrangements to meet them the first chance I got.

While in California, I had become interested in starting a collection of original oil paintings by unknown artists. One night, as I was leaving one of the apartments where I had promised to buy two paintings, I passed in front of the large picture window of the unit where the two new occupants had moved. I intended to take only a quick glance because I did not want to appear to be impolite or to get caught looking in. I nearly fell over my feet, and I'm sure my mouth dropped open, for inside that apartment was the skinny blonde I had observed unpacking the car, and also the most beautiful girl I had ever seen. I couldn't take my eyes off her. I smiled and waved, and nearly popped the buttons off the green uniform I was wearing.

The skinny blonde came over to the window and opened it wide enough to introduce herself and her roommate. The blonde was Ann and the other girl standing in the rear of the room was Ruth. They had just finished eating dinner. Ann asked me if I would like to come in and have some leftovers. Naturally, I said "No." Naturally, she asked again. Naturally, I said "Yes, I'd hate to see the food go to waste."

4

Ruth went into the kitchen and got a plate and some utensils while I sat down in the dining room. By this time I had forgotten how awkward I felt. I was totally engrossed in staring at this most captivating person. Ruth had the most gorgeous, penetrating large brown eyes perfectly accenting her long, curly, brown hair which was drawn into a ponytail behind her head. She had flawless skin and a perfectly proportioned body that would be the envy of many women and the admiration of most men. While she served me curried rice and chicken, I sat in awe of this young lady. I babbled something about my interest in painting, and with that Ruth politely excused herself to get something from the bedroom. When she returned to the dining room she brought a large artist's sketch pad. Ruth had aspirations of becoming a painter.

After dinner, we both looked through her sketch pad and talked about her artistic talents and drawings. Because I wanted to impress her with an oil painting, I excused myself, went to my apartment nearby, and brought back a nude painting of "Eve in the Garden of Eden," which I had recently purchased.

In a few minutes, I was showing off my cultured side, proudly admiring the painting with Ruth. I felt I was favorably impressing Ruth, so I didn't dare say I was drunk when I purchased that painting which hung behind a bar in Monterey. We talked about everything and nothing that evening. It was so simple and refined; it was beautiful. Later we watched *The Tonight Show* with Johnny Carson as well as part of *The Late, Late Show*. I left that night knowing I wanted to spend all my free time with this person.

From that time on, I made it a point to stop by to see Ruth right after work. The day didn't pass quickly enough. I wanted to get home as soon as possible to bask in her warm smile, a big hug, and a tender kiss.

One night, when I returned to my apartment after our usual visit, I was awakened by a pounding at the front door. I opened the door and there stood Ruth shivering and shaking. One of her old boyfriends had called and threatened her. She wanted to know if she could stay the night.

"Stay the night?" I thought to myself.

"Certainly. You may stay tonight and every other night you wish."

From that evening on, we spent entire weeks and months together enjoying each other's company. A walk down the beach became a lasting event. I was proud to be in her company and loved the opportunity to show her off. I loved the way she would fend off the stares of gawking men as she strolled down the beach. Because I couldn't keep my hands off her, shopping for groceries was a challenge to her ingenuity to avoid creating a scene. Motorcycle riding throughout the foothills of Pacific Grove became a cavalcade of colors and feelings. A gift from her was a thought of love. A dinner for two with candles, fine wine and exquisite china in a seafood restaurant overlooking San Francisco Bay was equally romantic to a hamburger and a coke at a sleazy, roadside stand.

No matter what we did or where we went, there was never a harsh word spoken between the two of us. Every day I would be amazed at her genuine kindness that made me feel complete.

I was the rough, cold, calculating, ambitious Army officer that no one dared to cross a second time. It was said of me, "He could watch a man bleed to death and not feel a thing." Ruth was my alter ego — the other side of me I left behind a long time ago. She was the child in me. She played herself while I seemed to be playing a role.

My time in the Army was rapidly coming to a close. I talked about my future plans in civilian life and, at Ruth's urging, I decided to apply to a graduate business school. I applied to and was accepted by

Oklahoma City University for the fall semester.

When the time came for me to leave, I treated the occasion with no emotion, caring or feeling. The day before I left, I met Ruth at the bank where she worked and took her out to lunch. At our farewell luncheon, my callous attitude showed its true colors. I talked about my leaving as easily as I could talk about changing a pair of shoes. I leaned over and coldly told Ruth to write when she got a chance. I told her I didn't write letters, and not to expect any from me. She burst into tears. Although I had never seen her cry before, the tears did not bother me. As a result, I spent my last night in California not with Ruth, but getting drunk with a motorcycle buddy.

At the airport the next morning, I felt very alone for the first time in my life. I had a sick, empty feeling in the pit of my stomach. I hoped to catch a last glimpse of Ruth seeing me off, but she was nowhere in sight.

When I arrived in Oklahoma City, I quickly registered for my courses and found an apartment right across from the campus. In spite of what I had said to Ruth about not writing, I wrote a letter telling her I had arrived safely and had rented an apartment. Within a couple of days I got a letter from her, wishing me well in my studies and saying she was leaving immediately for Europe.

I spent the next two months trying, in utter frustration, to carry on correspondence with her as she traveled throughout Europe. Soon I found that I was unable to study. It was then I learned, for the first time, I was in love.

I did not quite know what to say or do, but I knew I missed her terribly, in words and feelings that are difficult to describe. Unable to live without her, I sent her a letter asking her to marry me. I knew it would have been better if I had asked her three months earlier. But I had not known then that I was in love with her. She wrote back and asked me if I was sure.

"Sure, I'm sure," I thought to myself when I read the letter. I was never so sure of anything in my entire life. I ached at the thought of her not being at my side.

Soon my life and my studies became unbearable. One night I put down my books and said to myself, "I've got to get away and start doing something besides sitting here." I thought I had better start preparing for her return, as well as my career, by starting to work on a childhood dream of becoming a land developer. "After all," I thought, "I would have to someday support the both of us, and I couldn't study in school without Ruth by my side."

That same night, I made plans to move to Atlanta, because of the rapid real estate development which that city was then experiencing. Within five days, I dropped out of school and was winging my way to a new adventure. When I got to Atlanta, I stayed in a downtown hotel for a couple of days. During the first day, I walked around the city looking for a more permanent place to live. In one section of the city, I saw a stately three-story mansion that I was sure Ruth and I would someday share. The property was lined with tall shade trees which were just turning their fall colors. It was, I presumed, in one of the more exclusive sections of the city.

The next day, I scanned the local newspapers' help wanted sections and found an ad for a real estate salesperson. I called and made an appointment with a real estate broker who was situated a little to the north of the city. When I met him the next day, he appeared to be eager to see me and, more importantly, was willing to take me on as a salesman. He told me I would first have to obtain a license to sell property, and I needed enough money to tide me over until I collected my first sale's commission. We agreed that, by spring, I would have to satisfy both requirements.

I returned to the hotel elated at having been so fortunate.

The next afternoon, I found a small efficiency apartment across from the park in the center of the city. The building itself reminded me of an Army barracks. The apartment had a very small kitchen and a living room which doubled as a bedroom. I did not have any furniture, so I used a large packing crate as a bed. It was rather primitive, but I didn't care — I was in love.

One of my neighbors was kind enough to offer me any assistance I might need. I took him up on his offer and asked if he had a typewriter that I could use to type a new resumé which I hoped to use to get a position with one of the local accounting firms. I was employed by a Wall Street accounting firm before being drafted into the Army. As I sat typing the resumé, he told me about his life. He said, "One day I grew tired of the parade of life and quit my job. Now, I'm just an interested observer."

He talked about the Greek philosophers and their views about life. I was really in too much of a hurry to listen carefully, but I remember telling him I would rather be in the parade.

Armed with a resumé and a listing of certified

public accounting firms from a telephone book, I located one firm which was close by. I paid an unannounced visit. At my first stop I was referred to another firm which, in turn, referred me to still another, the latter being one of the largest accounting firms in Atlanta.

There, because of my previous accounting experience, I was more than welcomed by Mr. Andrews, the managing partner. He hired me that same day, and outlined my duties as a staff auditor. I was handed an employee policy manual and told my starting salary. It was not quite up to the offer of re-employment I had received from my former employers in New York City, but I reasoned that I could count heavily on the overtime pay, which was sure to come during the tax season that lay just ahead. I would use the proceeds to finance my real estate job coming up in the spring.

I became an accepted member of both the firm and the Andrews family. I even attended a reception given in honor of Mr. Andrews' daughter who was soon to be married.

The firm I had joined was a close family operation. It seemed everyone was related. Three of the five partners were brothers. Two sisters, who had not spoken to one another in thirty years outside of work, were also part of the ruling clan. The staff was more than willing to help a newcomer learn the ropes. Tales were told about the long hours I would soon be expected to keep. Throughout the upcoming tax season, twelve-hour work days would not be uncommon during a seven-day work week.

Characteristically, the first of the year marks the beginning of a very busy season with accounting firms. It appeared that this firm was no exception. The staff spent long hours preparing reports for year-end and tax deadlines. The long hours were not welcomed in most firms, but the over-time pay was certainly looked upon with great relish. This firm's manual said I would be paid at time-and-a-half for hours worked in excess of forty hours per week.

One weekday evening, out of the clear blue, I received a call from Mr. Bernstein, a commercial land developer who had learned of my interest in real estate. He called inviting me down to his office to speak about the possibility of joining his firm. I was gruff with him on the phone because my plans were already made to join the real estate brokerage firm early in the spring. However, I thought it would not hurt if I visited with him.

I met him later in the week at his office, which was located in one of the more prestigious office complexes in Atlanta. Mr. Bernstein talked about the time he arrived in Atlanta with only twenty dollars in his pocket. He told me that he was very successful. "Successful" was an understatement. His firm was responsible for developing one of the largest shopping complexes in the South. Right now he had more ambitious plans and was in the process of expanding his staff. Mr. Bernstein wanted to know if I might be interested in joining his firm. I told him I would consider his offer. He then asked me what I was interested in earning per year. I had never given it much thought, but I figured when playing ball with the big guys, and they ask *you* to play with *them*, tell them what they want to hear. I almost choked when I said, "Seventy thousand." I thought it was a ridiculous answer. Not to be outdone, he told me one hundred thousand was not out of the question. But he told me that I must first decide exactly what I wanted to accomplish in the real estate business. I couldn't help but think that if he saw my apartment and the shipping crate I called my bed, this entire conversation would be absurd.

Don Bernstein, as he preferred to be called, also

asked me to find out the names of the three individuals who ran Atlanta. I thought it was a cute test. When I got back to the accounting firm office, I had the names of the three men in fifteen minutes, from a knowledgeable staff. They were in the dark about my plans for the spring, but were aware of my relationship with Ruth, who was still traveling throughout Europe.

I immediately started to formalize my plans about what I wanted to accomplish in real estate. I saw a company that would build homes, shopping centers, schools, recreational centers, and move horizontally across the entire real estate spectrum. I also envisioned a company that would move vertically to take over sources of supply. During the day, I was an auditor. At night I worked out my plans for a real estate conglomerate.

Contrary to the published policy manual, I soon learned via the grapevine that the accounting firm had never paid overtime but gave Christmas bonuses instead. This did not sit well with me, especially since I had already received a bonus at the Christmas party, along with a raise. Perturbed at this unforeseen development, I asked for clarification of the firm's policy and was told that no overtime wages would be paid. As far as I was concerned, no overtime pay meant no work.

On the first Saturday I was scheduled for overtime, I told the accountant in charge that I would not show up. It must have been the first time someone had ever said no to him because he bought me lunch at the Country Club and tried to talk me into joining him at work on Saturday. His plan did not work.

Back at the office the following Monday, he asked me why I did not show up on Saturday. When I told him, "No pay, no work," he took off like a gray-haired, stoop-shouldered kid who was going to tell your mother that you stole a cookie, and marched right to Mr. Andrews' office.

The office was now abuzz with rumor and conflict. I had declared an unofficial war. I told the other accountants that all other professional accounting firms paid overtime. I told them they were being cheated, and I explained why, by statute and policy, people who endured long hours deserved overtime pay.

By the end of the week, I had not heard how management was going to deal with me. I had decided to stay until spring and then take the firm to court to sue them for overtime wages. Some of the other accountants heeded my advice and started looking for opportunities elsewhere.

I was soon sent out of the office on a one week field audit. As soon as I returned, I learned I was scheduled to be sent out on another field audit of a clothing manufacturer in southern Georgia. This audit was scheduled for two weeks. Just before I left, I received a letter from Ruth stating that she was returning to California the following week and had decided to put an end to our relationship.

Surprised at this turn of event, and hurt beyond measure, I wrote to her parents' California address to say that I would be out to see her in two weeks. This was the scheduled end of the field audit.

I told the accountant in charge that I was going to fly out and finally see Ruth, and ask her to marry me. He understood and said it would be a good idea if I worked through the first weekend to make sure the audit would be finished on time. That weekend, the accountant in charge went home to Atlanta, and I stayed on the job.

When he returned on Monday morning, he said that I would have to stay on the job right through the next weekend. I reminded him of my plans and told him that under no circumstances would I stay on the job when I was going to see Ruth. He told me he would have to clear this with the head office. When he returned from making the phone call, I was told to report to Mr. Andrews' office that afternoon.

"Damn," I thought to myself, "I've gone and done it now. Five will get you ten I'm going to get fired. This is the way they are going to deal with me and my fight to get paid for overtime work."

On the way back to Atlanta, I decided I'd better see Don Bernstein right away. I would talk to him about my plans for a real estate conglomerate, and with any luck at all, be hired right on the spot. Then I would be able to walk into Mr. Andrews' office and quit in style.

When I got to Don Bernstein's office, I learned Don had just returned from Switzerland but would still see me. We started our conversation where we had left off at our last meeting. I told him about my plans, and it was soon obvious that was not what he wanted to hear. My plans and his plans were definitely not the same. The more we talked to each other, the more it became apparent that what he offered and what I wanted were two different things. He wanted a commercial real estate person, and I wanted to start a conglomerate. Three times, Don asked me to change my plans and join his firm. Three times, I refused. His last question to me was, "Do you know what you really want to do?" I lied when I said, "I am really sure." When I left his office I caught myself having second and third thoughts about what I had just done. I turned down a golden opportunity and was soon to face the prospects of being fired.

I caught a taxi up to the main office and arrived just before five o'clock. I was ushered into Mr. Andrew's office. He said simply, "We do not think that you would be happy to continue your employment here. So, I'm asking for your resignation. You will be paid up through today, along with severance pay and any overtime pay you feel is due."

I tried to put up a good front by asking for a letter of reference to indicate that I was being let go because of a dispute over pay and not because of any professional shortcomings. Mr. Andrews said he would see to it. I was, by this time, becoming completely unglued and the cracks were beginning to show in my usually cool exterior. I walked back into the staff room to pick up my things and mumbled something about how much this job meant to Ruth and me.

I left the office with my pay check in hand and turned up the street in a daze, not really believing what had just happened and not really knowing where I was going. I grabbed the first bus that came by and felt someone was playing a mean trick on me; I wanted to cry. I wanted out of the parade. I buried my head in shame. The fight was out of me. I was broken in spirit. I would have been grateful if the earth had opened up and swallowed me whole. I had, in the space of two weeks, been fired from a job, turned down a fantastic job offer three times, and lost the only girl I cared for beyond measure. When I finally looked up, the bus was empty except for the bus driver and me. He asked me where I was going. I told him where I lived. He told me I was on the wrong bus.

"That does it," I thought to myself. "I need time to put my life back in order. I'm going back to school in Oklahoma, via California."

Ruth called that night from California, she woke me from a sound sleep to tell me she was going to see her brother and wouldn't be able to see me. I tried to explain what had just happened, but the words never came. Now, my world was shattered. I prayed that I would not wake up in the morning.

Morning came. The day went. Evening came. The evening went. I did not stir for two days. "No one cares," I thought. I was finally out of the parade.

On the morning of the third day I grew hungry, and my spirits were beginning to be revived. I was still determined to return to Oklahoma via California and start all over again. I resolved never again to be the last person to know I was in love. I reasoned that had I known about "being in love," all these tragedies could have been avoided.

I flew to California on Monday and returned to Pacific Grove where I thought Ruth would be staying. I looked up her old roommate, Ann, and learned that Ruth was living with her parents just outside San Francisco and had started working for a bank.

Ironically, I stayed the night with my old motorcycle-riding buddy whom I had gotten drunk with the night before I left for Oklahoma. Early the next day, I arrived at Ruth's parent's apartment, but no one was home. I spent the rest of the day going from bank to bank, hoping to surprise Ruth at work. I couldn't find the right bank.

So I returned to their apartment and waited in the lobby until Ruth walked in about a half an hour later with her mother. When Ruth saw me, she immediately looked down at the floor, and I knew for sure that it was over between us. We talked for a while. She told me I was no longer the man in her life. I stayed the night in a motel and returned the next day to give it one more try. I did not succeed.

When I arrived back in Oklahoma City, I found that my baggage had been misdirected to Mexico City. I quickly rented an apartment and went inside.

As far as Ruth was concerned, my affair of love was over. I was left quite alone in this world to face the ordeal of depression, of unrequited love, and of self-hatred. I hated myself completely for what I had done. There was no way out as far as I was concerned.

The god that I prayed to at night did not seem to listen or care, and I was beyond all help. There was to be no recovery. I was doomed and fated to be alone. The more helpless and pitiful I became, the more I turned to prayer. God would help and send me an understanding, although an understanding was not what I wanted. I wanted Ruth. I was the valiant bull crawling into a corner to die from deep, terrible wounds. Again, I wanted out of this world. I didn't want to face another day without Ruth. Once again, I went to bed and did not want to face another lonely day.

When I awoke I took endless, aimless walks through space and time. I hated to see happy couples in love. My heart was torn at the sight of them. Gutless, I returned to sleep. This was my escape from reality, this world of sleep. Sleep was nothing and meaningless, and that meant something to me: I ceased to exist. God would and could, I thought, return Ruth to me. Powerless to help myself, I turned to him.

I became sick. Fever racked my body. I was glad in a way. Maybe she would hear of my plight and come to my rescue. "Wake up! Catch hold of yourself!" I thought to myself. "There's no one now. You must take care of yourself."

Finally I got out of bed, dressed and walked down the street into a doctor's office to take care of my illness. While I waited I reviewed my speech; "It started two days ago. I don't know what it's from. Could you give me some pills to relieve the fever?" The nurse told me the doctor would see me now. As soon as I saw the doctor, I felt silly and embarrassed at being there. Even as he examined me and took my temperature, I felt a compulsion to talk about my recent tragedies. He was a middle-aged man who wore a white shirt and a skinny string tie. His stethoscope hung loosely around his neck and he had two pens in his shirt pocket. He reminded me of a doctor who my mother took me to see when I was young. Before he said anything, I came to my senses and apologized for wasting his time. He pushed my comments aside and told me I was running a slight temperature. He told me that it was nothing to worry about and that I would be okay in a couple of days.

There was a chill in the air as I walked out of his office. I began to assess my situation. I told myself to go out and get a job. The economic realities of life were going to catch up with me if I did not get a job quickly.

The next day, I dressed in my favorite dark-blue suit, which finally was returned from Mexico City. I headed for downtown Oklahoma City. I went to an employment agency that billed itself as a management recruiting firm. There, I spoke to a recruiter who asked me if I would like to sell computers. He thought that with my outgoing personality and my accounting experience, I would be a good salesman. "Sure, why not?" I said. He called the firm and lined me up for an interview with the branch manager that same afternoon.

It was a good feeling to be wanted, even if it was only for a job interview. I had plenty of experience in job interviews in my senior year of college. When I finished talking with the branch manager, he was eager to hire me. However, he told me I would have to meet with the computer division sales manager who was out of town on business for a couple of days.

When I left the sales office, I was sure that I had secured the job. I stopped by church to give thanks. It was so peaceful and quiet in there. I loved the feeling of solitude. It had been ages since I visited church on a day other than Sunday. I resolved then to renew my acquaintance with god by prayer. This was the start of a nightly practice. I never told anyone I prayed at night because I felt embarrassed at what people might think. I prayed in private.

I prayed that Ruth, I, and my family would be taken care of. I asked for guidance. I wanted to know why these things had happened to me. Why did he allow it to happen? I had a burning desire to understand. I relied upon "him" to square things away and right everything in my life.

Before I heard from the computer sales manager, I wrote several long, rambling letters to Ruth, expressing my devotion to her. I heaped promises upon promises, remorse upon remorse. I was starting to get things out of my system. Hopeless as it seemed, I felt I was doing something about my situation.

I soon heard from the sales manager, who said that I had the sales position and should report to the branch office on Monday. Shortly thereafter, he said, I would be sent to Rochester, New York, for a data processing sales course.

Walking into any new employment situation brings a certain tingle of excitement. On Monday, I was warmly greeted and shown the premises. I was introduced to the people with whom I would be working. I attached myself to one of the salesmen who was about my own age. He told me what was expected of me, and talked about the good times I would have in Rochester during the next month. There were the usual exaggerated stories about loose women and drinking parties.

He told me I was expected to bone up for a data processing entrance exam that was going to be given to me as soon as I arrived in Rochester. I was shown my desk and told to review all the prepared material about the product line. I was told that usually there is at least a six-month training period, but, because of the critical need for computer sales, I would be sent to the school in two weeks.

When I arrived in Rochester, I flunked the entrance exam with flying colors. But, because of the short time I was with the company, I could remain at the center. I was happy to be in a new situation, and the spirit rubbed off. I studied hard for the subsequent exams, and, although I did not graduate at the top of my class, at least I did not flunk any more tests.

By the third week of the course, the routine became a grind. Classes do have a way of becoming very boring very quickly. I would let my mind wander occasionally and would catch myself daydreaming. Often, I would flash back to some beautiful interlude with Ruth and then return to the course instructor's presentation.

During one lecture session, I was sitting directly in front of the instructor, who was an immaculately dressed, well-spoken, former computer salesman. Al and I hit it right off. We would trade comments back and forth between classes. On one occasion, when I was not paying attention to what Al was saying, I noticed that he was scratching his earlobe at the same time I was scratching my ear. This observation would have passed as any other casual observation, and I doubt whether I would have placed much importance to an ear-scratching episode, except that I caught myself scratching my ear again, and a few seconds later, I noticed Al was scratching his earlobe again.

I had always been concerned about whether I was a leader or a follower, and I decided this was a case of "monkey see, monkey do." The only thing I was concerned about was who scratched first. For the hell of it, I pulled on my nose. Al followed suit. Surprise of surprises! Something was at work that I did not know anything about, and I became intrigued at the possibilities. I scratched at the back of my head, and Al did it, too. He did what I did.

If someone had a movie camera, this episode would have been priceless to record because neither of us were fully aware of what was going on until I pulled my nose. He did it, too. I gloated at the idea of being the leader in this instance.

Things became a lot more interesting at school after that. I put meanings on any of the gestures that I saw the teachers or students making. I was soon able to predict when a gesture was going to be repeated. I remember one student in particular sitting at the front of the class with his back towards us. He was in the middle of giving a demonstration on correct data entry procedures. Every time Al would make a correction, the student would pick up his feet which were, up until the correction, positioned flat on the floor. Afterwards, I knew that every time a correction was given this student was going to cross his legs under the chair.

I soon began to notice gestures that were constantly being repeated by different people in the same types of situations. Crossed arms meant disagreement. An index finger pointed to the ear meant the person was listening. Fingers in front of the mouth meant "Be careful what you say." Scratching the throat indicated that you wanted to say something.

I was fast learning more about body language than computer sales procedures. When I returned to Oklahoma City, I used my new-found knowledge to talk a comptroller into letting our firm conduct a computer installation feasibility study of his firm. It was easy. I didn't know enough about sales or computers to really sell him on our system's advantages, but I did know enough about body language to reverse my field whenever he crossed his arms to show me his silent disagreement with anything I said. When I saw him cross his arms, I would say anything I could think of to the contrary, and the comptroller would then uncross his arms, thereby showing me silent agreement.

It would be more than a year before I would return to study body language. In the meantime, I returned to graduate school night classes on a full-time basis. During that year I became so engrossed in school and work that I rarely thought about Ruth. However, I did call her, ostensibly to ask for an address of a mutual friend. She did not know his address, but I did learn that Ruth was happily looking forward to moving to Hawaii. That was the last I heard about Ruth — my first real love and the woman who had such a profound effect on my life.

Chapter Two
QUIET THOUGHTS

I have begun my story of cancer cure with my affair of love with Ruth because were it not for that drama, this story might not have been written. Prior to this, I took life as it came. I never wondered about life. I left explanations to theologians, psychologists, and philosophers. But the events and circumstances surrounding my loss of Ruth's love compelled me to change my ways.

I now included, along with my commercial interests, an interest in religion, psychology, and philosophy. I used all these disciplines to provide explanations wherever possible. When these ways of thinking did not satisfy my intense desire to learn about myself, I used the resources of my own mind.

I now feel it's necessary to write this story because of what I have learned by using the resources of my own mind. I feel it is important in relating this story of a cancer cure to create a believable atmosphere, yet one which will invite testing. Only then, after testing the validity of the assertions, can a determination be made of the accuracy of this story.

The loss of Ruth's love in my life created an intense desire to learn about myself. I wanted to know the moment I was again in love, not to find out three months later. This intense desire for self awareness opened up channels of the mind that I never knew existed. I did not know, for example, that each person has a personal answer bank. This answer bank may be called upon any time an individual wants answers to personal questions.

My realization that each person has a personal answer bank was an evolutionary process, rather than something that happened overnight. Through the years, I began to rely less and less upon ready-made answers to questions from organized religion, psychology and philosophy, and to rely more upon answers from this personal answer bank.

As it happened, though, I relied upon ready made childhood beliefs to accept the fact that Ruth and I had separated. I accepted my separation from Ruth as being part of god's will. I had become lost in a sea of personal questions, which I was determined to have answered. Chief among these questions was "Why were Ruth and I separated?" I was determined to learn from the god I thought to be "all-knowing" the reasons behind this separation. These reasons I thought could be learned from god once I established a line of communication through prayer. I expected my prayers to be answered because god provided for all our needs, and I certainly needed answers.

This expectation that my question to god would be answered carried over into other questions that I asked, but not in prayers. And the attitude that my questions would be answered opened up channels for information that I never had access to before.

I was puzzled over my own body language and asked myself this question: "Why do I rub my shoulder?" This response came to mind: *BECAUSE YOU FEEL LONELY*. Because first replies like this came in the form of unspoken words, phrases, or sentences, I called them quiet thoughts. "Quiet thoughts" is the term I use to describe all answers to questions that originated from inner sources. Later, when I learned that quiet thoughts were not necessarily quiet, I would also use the term "projections" to help me identify answers that originated from inner sources.

The first term I used, "quiet thoughts," helped me understand something about the nature of these responses to my questions. When I asked myself, "How does rubbing help me?" this reply came to mind: *BY RUBBING AND CARESSING YOURSELF, YOU ARE SAYING YOU ARE LOVED AND NOT ALONE.* I knew I had never heard or read about this explanation for rubbing before. Therefore, the explanation had to come from some inner source of knowledge. This inner source of knowledge I would later identify as a part of the mind called an answer bank.

By using the term quiet thoughts, I was reminded to be alert for these responses to my personal questions or I might miss them. When I asked myself why I felt lonely, this reply came to mind: *BECAUSE YOU FEEL UNWANTED AND UNLOVED.* I knew, unless I was alert for the quiet thoughts, the replies might escape me.

While I continued to ask myself questions about my own body language and to learn explanations through quiet thoughts, I discovered something else about quiet thoughts. Quiet thoughts, as I've already noted, were not always quiet. If you listened closely to your own conversations or the conversations of others, you could hear quiet thoughts being verbalized. I used the term "projections" to help me understand that answers to all questions a person asked himself that originated from their inner sources could be projected outside the person. Because my first awareness of these responses was in the form of spoken words, I called them projections. Just as you had to be alert for quiet thoughts, you had to be alert for projections in a normal conversation or you might miss them.

For example, when I told a friend to pay more attention to what his body language meant, I realized my advice to him was a projection. I realized that I, not my friend, should pay more attention to my own body language. I projected onto my friends what courses of action I should follow. Later, I realized that we all project answers to our self-directed questions when we talk about our friends.

My first real-life observation of this projection phenomenon is a good example. It was made at a poolside party in Oklahoma City, during a conversation with a manufacturing executive who ran a plastics company in the same city. The executive, Charles McCoy, became interested in joining the unofficial power structure of Oklahoma City. According to Charles, the men who really ran the city worked behind the scenes. One member was the head of a large oil company, another was the publisher of the daily newspaper, and the last member was an official in a church organization. These men, according to Charles, decided who would be selected to run for public office. Charles wanted to become a part of this unofficial power structure. He tried to join all the right clubs and was a member of many fraternal organizations. We passed the time talking about my graduate business courses and his business ventures for about an hour. Then Charles turned to me and said, "Tom, you shouldn't worry about joining the Quail Creek Country Club, because those who run the city will not accept you. You have to be born into the unofficial power structure of the city. Your kids would stand a better chance."

What Charles was saying to me was so far away from my interests that I thought his advice was absurd. I was an unmarried university student who had no aspirations of joining either the official or unofficial power structure of Oklahoma City. Later that same night, I tried to figure out how Charles ever got the idea that I was worried about joining the Quail Creek Country Club. Then it dawned on me; Charles was talking to himself out loud. I was being used by

Charles as his personal sounding board. He was projecting what he should do onto my personality. Somehow Charles could better listen to himself when he heard the words of advice he gave me.

These words of advice or answers to self-directed questions I called projections. Charles had been worrying about whether or not to join the country club and this was the reply from his own personal answer bank. A sense of personal direction was but one attribute of the type of answers that could be learned from this inner source.

I confirmed my first observation of projections by many other observations. I found myself listening more closely to people whenever they talked. I was listening for projections that provided a sense of direction. I was surprised at the number of times during the day that this phenomenon could be observed.

I was talking one day with a girl named JoAnn, who was trying to decide if she should continue dating a boyfriend. JoAnn talked freely of her doubts and fears, and of the good and bad points about dating Stan. After she finished talking through her situation, JoAnn seemed ready to turn her attention to another subject. But then JoAnn spoke these words of advice "You know, Tom, you should give the relationship with the girl you are dating more time to develop." It is at this point in the conversation that I decided to play back for JoAnn her projection onto my personality about what she should do. I was careful to use the exact words JoAnn used in her projection. I would neither add to nor subtract anything from the projection. Nor did I substitute my own words, which might confuse the issue or the objectified direction JoAnn was giving herself. I soon found out that the best advice I could give to someone was to listen carefully for their own projections or objectified answers when they talked about their friends. I used the term "objectified answers" to point out that a person could identify and examine answers outside him or herself.

By the end of my first year of graduate school, I asked questions about my personality that I expected to be answered through quiet thoughts. I also developed the habit of asking questions at night before I went to sleep and of paying close attention to new ideas I had the next day. For example, if I asked "Why am I now just beginning to understand people?" sometime during the next day I would have this quiet thought: *WHEN YOU SPEND YOUR DAY TRYING TO THINK UP WAYS TO UNDERSTAND, AN UNDERSTANDING*

WILL BE YOURS BECAUSE OF DESIRE.

During the summer months away from school, I would spend hours talking with acquaintances about what little I knew about projections and a great deal of time talking about body language. It was fun. I loved the game aspect of trying to figure out particular gestures and movements. People loved to hear someone talk about what their body movements meant. I relied upon my good memory for quiet thoughts about body language to help me during these conversations. By now I had become familiar with both quiet thoughts and projection-type material. It may be easier for a reader, who would like to understand what a quiet thought is like, if you say the following sentence out loud: "Body language is an unwritten language." Now say the same sentence to yourself silently. When you say the sentence silently to yourself, that is what a quiet thought is like. When you say the sentence out loud, you see how easy it is to verbalize a quiet thought. I had developed a three-hour monologue on body language, based solely on quiet thoughts. But I soon tired of talking about body language. Instead, I became more interested in learning about projections.

I was intrigued at the possibility that there might

be more to projections than I originally thought. Subsequent observations about the projection phenomena would cause me to conclude that projections could be used as a valuable key to understanding something about another person quickly.

For instance, Mary Doe may be talking about her friend Peggy and say, "My friend Peggy is the most terrible gossip in town who never gets anything straight. Lately, Peggy's been in lots of trouble because she can't keep her big mouth shut. Peggy has got to learn to keep her big mouth shut for a change." Mary, in this instance, is saying that Mary, not Peggy, is a gossip who should learn to keep her mouth shut. Before reaching any objective conclusion about Peggy's personality, you would have to hear what Peggy thinks about her friends.

This reversal, of applying things we all say about our friends to ourselves, does not always work. But for now, I would like to broaden my definition of projections from "statements containing answers to self-directed questions" to now also include this new idea. The new idea is "Whenever we talk about our friends, we are talking about ourselves." I am sure that in most conversations almost anyone can find projections of another's personality. After you catch on to the game, which is very simple to play, I am sure you will be amazed at what people unwittingly say about themselves.

To the trained observer, the presence of projections is taken for granted in most conversations. What sometimes gives the trained observer trouble is putting a projection in proper perspective. For example, when John Doe is anxiously criticizing his friend Jerry and says, "Jerry is really a lazy man who would rather loaf around the house all day than put in an honest day's work," it might take time to put this projection into its proper perspective because John Doe is a hard worker who works hard to hide his own laziness from others and himself. In the example, John Doe is anxiously dealing with two opposing views of himself. Many cases of simple anxiety like this one may be cleared up by the person dealing successfully with the two opposing projections. How to deal with opposing beliefs will be discussed later.

Shortly after I learned about these parts of our everyday conversations that I called projections, I attempted to try and understand anything a person might say in a conversation to see what he might unwittingly reveal about his personality. I was also looking for the hidden meanings or innuendos behind words, which for the most part are just unobserved. In the example just given about John Doe, who was critical of his friend Jerry, the innuendo is obvious. John Doe should be critical about his own attitudes, not Jerry's supposed laziness. Generally, critics should point the finger of criticism at themselves.

With my newfound knowledge about projections, and with my new interest in trying to understand a person from anything he said during a conversation, I decided to test my resourcefulness by talking with people. It was not difficult to find people who were interested in these ideas. Conversations were my testing grounds for these new ideas. It may be that you have read these same ideas before, but I had never heard about them. I wanted to find out if I was correct or incorrect, and I figured the best way to learn about people was from people who would surely correct any misconceptions I had.

I made a game out of these tests. Although I never asked a friend outright if he would like to play the understanding game, I would just get around to the subject without ever saying what I was doing. I compared the game to a tennis match. The volley was the conversation. Points were scored when the opposing players could not refute what the other person had said. The object of the game was to disprove my statement that anything you say reveals something about your personality. You won the game when you disproved my statement. I won the game when I supported my statement by telling you something about yourself from something you said during the conversation.

Imagine for a moment that we have just met. We talk for about twenty minutes when I casually mention that whenever you say something, you unwittingly reveal something about your personality. In all likelihood you are going to choose your next words very carefully. You will try to answer my statement by saying something to disprove what I just said.

Your reply to me might go something like this: "That's a ridiculous statement. It just can't be true. You mean when I call a friend of mine a cheat, I'm a cheater. That isn't true, I'm not a cheater."

Now the burden of proof lies in my court. I was expected to back up what I just said or stop playing the game. In most instances, I loved the challenge of proving what I had just said. It was a game I enjoyed. I created the game, so I knew the game better than most beginning players. The first rule I had was to listen carefully to whatever a person said for some ammunition to throw back at him when the expected denial came. The denial usually came in the form of an example that almost always followed the general trend of the conversation we were having. The second rule was to be able to remember exactly what was said by the opponent.

In the example just given in which my opponent denied he was a cheater, I recalled that earlier in the conversation he had bragged about copying answers from another student during an exam. In ninety-nine instances out of a hundred, the expected denial proved my point and I won the game. When I reminded my opponent of what he said earlier, he smiled. When there was a smile, or a sudden silence, I had won the match.

The best defensive players say nothing. If the opposing player said nothing, he won the match.

I had other rules about the game I was playing. I only played singles matches. One-on-one was best because something might be said by the opponent which could prove embarrassing. He was more likely to admit to a fault in private than with other people around. I also only play this game with people who I thought could handle the situation. Sometimes I made a mistake and got violent verbal reactions. When this did happen, I backed down from what I said and he won by default.

All words used to describe another person do not always characterize the person speaking.

When it first came time for me to deal with my own projections, I was a sore sport. I didn't like the game. I didn't want to know anymore unwelcome things about myself than I had already learned through projections. I was the poor millionaire who worked hard to get where he was and then hated the money. Because I was only looking for my faults, my projections reflected this outlook. When I changed my attitude, I learned about my good points.

Changing some of my personality traits, or the unwelcome things I learned about myself through projections, was a different challenge altogether. The first method I used was rather primitive but effective nevertheless. I relied upon wishful thinking. When I projected that I was stubborn (and I did not like to be stubborn because I thought this was being close-minded), I would automatically wish I was open-minded. After a time, because my mental intention was properly channeled by effective wishful thinking, I changed my personality and became open-minded. The speed with which my personality traits changed varied in direct proportion to the amount of disgust I had with my projections. The more disgust, the more quickly I changed my personality. Sometime later, I would learn how to formalize my effective wishful thinking into a personality-trait-change process. I would write down the unwelcome trait I projected, and alongside I wrote the trait I wanted to acquire. Then I would form one or two simple sentences that objectified my wishful thinking into a clearly stated mental intention. Then, for a few minutes a day, I would dwell on my remarks that I had put down on paper. After I felt comfortable with my new trait, I would stop concentrating on the remarks. My new trait was achieved by accepting the new view I wanted and by getting rid of the old view. For example, when I wanted to deal with my "being stubborn" projection, the sentences I used were something like this: "My stubborn trait was a part of my personality. Now, in this new instance, I am open-minded."

Once I wanted to become a linguist (and I didn't have to deal with any doubts), I used this effective wishful thinking technique to convince myself that I was a linguist. I concentrated on this sentence: "I direct that I am now a linguist." I stopped concentrating on this objectified mental intention when

I found myself spending all my free time studying foreign languages. Eventually, it turned out that the new image I thought I wanted, which did result in a change of behavior, was not what I really wanted to become after all.

I don't worry about unwelcome projections now because I can use this effective wishful thinking technique to change my personality. Once you experiment and learn how quickly you can change your personality, you can have fun changing it to suit your own permanent requirements or just your temporary whims.

I continued my exploration of projections and quiet thoughts even more extensively than I ever anticipated. If, through quiet thoughts, I could both learn about my body language and have personal questions answered, I wondered if I could now project or verbalize answers to the problems I was facing.

If I was having a problem standing up in front of the class to give an oral report, could I solve this problem by using projections? My tests showed me that the answer bank, through either projections or quiet thoughts, does stand ready to answer all questions.

For example, sometime during the day I asked

myself, "How should I handle myself in front of the class in giving this report?" Then I added this direction: "I direct that I project the answer when I talk about a friend." I repeated this question and direction a few times to make sure that I had the proper mental intention, which would then trigger responses from the answer bank. Later in the day, when I thought out loud about my friend, I would offer to myself a solution for my fear of getting up in front of a class to speak. I said, "He would do a lot better at work (class) if he was better prepared to answer questions from his boss (teacher). Then Frank (I) would not be so scared to talk with his boss (teacher)." By substituting one word for another, the projection becomes a lot clearer. "I would do a lot better in giving oral reports if I was better prepared to answer questions from my teacher. Then I would not be so scared to talk in front of class." With a little practice, I was better able to identify examinable or objectified answers to my questions by means of these monologues.

However, I rarely used this projection problem-solving technique outside my own sphere of interest. Through a quiet thought, I had learned that my concern with social problems was a way to avoid my own personal problems. Consequently, I left the giant challenges of the day to the experts who were in a position to do something about difficult problems. However, in my master's degree thesis (or problem paper) I had to address myself to the question of unemployment because my paper was on an aspect of international financial management. I did not know how to treat the unemployment problem in my paper.

I considered for a long time many unacceptable social and economic solutions. As the deadline for the paper approached, I found myself debating this problem just before I went to sleep. In the morning I awoke with this quiet thought: *TAKE THE WORK THAT TWELVE DO AND DIVIDE IT AMONG THIRTEEN. LIKEWISE SHARE THE EARNINGS FOR TWELVE AMONG THIRTEEN. PROFITS AND COSTS REMAINING THE SAME. NOW IN AMERICA YOU SHARE EVERYTHING BUT THE WORK.*

I had never considered solving the unemployment problem in this manner before, but quiet thoughts had a way of coming up with the unexpected.

After I graduated from school, I worked during summer as a painter, and then I traveled extensively throughout Europe and the Near East. When I returned home to New York, I decided to start my own painting contracting company. By being self-employed, I could take time off whenever I wanted to travel. Following my second year of being self-employed, I lived for a time in Barbados, a small country off the coast of South America. Wherever I went, I talked about my ideas on human personality, projections, quiet thoughts, body language, changing your personality, problem-solving techniques, and each person's ability to solve all his own personal problems by using his own personal answer bank.

Because I loved to talk over these ideas with people, I decided to apply to a university for a teaching position. It did not dawn on me to ask myself what I should do to get a teaching position. I just decided to ask myself three difficult questions. The answers, I hoped, would impress the university officials enough to hire me as a teacher.

On one hand, I was convinced of my god-given talent to answer these three difficult questions, but, on the other hand, I did not know what to do with my learning, as later events will point out. One of the three questions was related to physics, the next was related to religion, and the last was related to medicine. I asked and received answers for the first two questions, but these quiet thoughts do not relate to my story. The last question was "What is a method that may be used to find a cure for cancer?" I have edited this lengthy quiet thought slightly and have also added several subsequent quiet thoughts for the purpose of continuity: *ANIMALS WHO HAVE THE DISEASE OR WHO HAVE BEEN INJECTED WITH THE DISEASE SHOULD BE INSTRUCTED THAT YOU WOULD LIKE THEM TO LEAD YOU TO A NATURAL CURE. ANIMALS WILL UNDERSTAND IN THEIR MANNER WHAT YOU WOULD LIKE THEM TO DO. ALLOW THEM COMPLETE FREEDOM TO SEEK THE CURE THEY ARE ALREADY AWARE OF, OR WILL LEARN, AMONG THE NATURAL HERBS AND MINERALS OF THIS EARTH.*

I was sitting at my desk at home when I got this quiet thought to my third question, the one on medicine, the question posed. I was a little alarmed because of the immediacy of the reply. I also wondered where to start the hunt, even though I had never considered using animals in this way before. Later that same night, I asked, "Where do you start the hunt?" just before I went to sleep. In the morning, I had this quiet thought: *ONE AREA TO START THE RESEARCH IS SALINAS, CALIFORNIA. FOLLOWING THIS ANIMAL'S FOOTSTEPS, YOU WILL FIND A*

CURE FOR CANCER.

That night, when I sat down at my desk, the quiet thoughts continued to flow: *THE KNOWLEDGE YOU SEEK IS ALREADY AVAILABLE TO US. THIS WAY IS BETTER BECAUSE OF THE SYMBOLIC VALUES WHICH WOULD BE LOST WERE WE TO USE ANOTHER WAY.*

THE DISCOVERY OF A CANCER CURE BY AN ANIMAL WILL SYMBOLICALLY STAND FOR OUR ONENESS WITH THE UNIVERSE AND THE ANIMALS OF THE WORLD AND SHOW THE SACREDNESS OF EVEN ONE MOUSE. THIS WILL SERVE TO STOP THE UNNEEDED SLAUGHTER OF THE ANIMALS IN OUR LABS BY MEN WHO HAVE GROWN DEAF TO THEIR CRIES. IT WILL BE THE FOOTSTEPS HEARD AROUND THE WORLD.

NATURAL DRUGS ARE NOT A SUBSTITUTE FOR THE NATURAL HEALING PROCESSES OF THE BODY, WHICH ARE FAR SUPERIOR. BUT IT WILL SERVE THOSE WHO, BECAUSE OF THEIR BELIEFS, SEE DRUGS AS THE CURE. THE NATURAL CURE RESTS OUTSIDE THE CAGES AND THE BUILDINGS THAT SERVE TO CONTAIN OUR CONSCIOUS KNOWLEDGE AND RESTRAIN ANIMALS FROM SHOWING US THE WAY.

REMEMBER PENICILLIN. I HAVE HYPHENATED THE WORD RE-SEARCH TO POINT OUT THAT THE KNOWLEDGE YOU SEEK IS ALREADY AVAILABLE TO US.

The following are the subsequent quiet thoughts I have added to the original reply for the purpose of continuity: *WILD AND DOMESTIC ANIMALS ARE BOTH EQUIPPED TO SEEK OUT NATURAL CURES. WILD ANIMALS WILL PERFORM BETTER BECAUSE INSTINCTIVE BEHAVIORAL PATTERNS HAVE NOT BEEN ALTERED. BEFRIENDING OF WILD ANIMALS WILL HELP TO DEVELOP NECESSARY LEVELS OF COMMUNICATIONS. THE TRAINING OF PERSONS SHOULD PROCEED TO ENABLE THESE PERSONS TO BE RECEPTIVE TO ANIMAL COMMUNICATIONS NOT NOW POSSIBLE. THIS WILL MAKE IT POSSIBLE TO LEARN THE INFORMATION YOU REQUIRE DIRECTLY FROM THE ANIMALS WITHOUT THE NEED FOR TRACKING.*

I wrote in a letter to the dean of a well-known medical school the original quiet thoughts in response to my question, "What is a method that may be used to find a cure for cancer?" After I mailed the letter, which also contained the quiet thoughts on the physics and religion questions, I thought about what I had just written to a complete stranger. I decided that no one was ever going to believe me.

The dean did not answer my letter.

Chapter Three
THE CURE

Although I was able to deal with the many things I learned through quiet thoughts about my personality, when it came time for me to deal with learnings outside my direct sphere of interest, I did not know what to do. So, my next step in dealing with this new method of using animals to find cures for diseases was to include this idea, along with other assorted ideas that I had begun to collect, in a notebook.

For some time afterwards, I devoted myself to developing further applications of the projection and quiet thoughts theory. I was still relying on a Christian folklore to explain my abilities to answer questions. This mythology says god meets all our needs. I updated this folklore to include not only our material needs but also our knowledge requirements.

I was expanding my horizons by using the quiet thought material as a practical means of solving everyday problems. I loved to talk about my interests to acquaintances who were interested in learning about my new found way of learning about themselves. My horizons were further expanded one evening when I happened to meet a girl named Karin, who suggested that I read a book called Seth Speaks by Jane Roberts. I began reading the book, which contained a number of the same ideas that I had already included in my notebook.

One of these ideas, which I had already been developing, was explored in that book. It was that man has a bank of answers which may be called upon within himself. It was also suggested by the author that a bank of answers exists outside man, which also may be utilized. Because I had already proven to my satisfaction that man has a bank of answers within himself which he may call upon, I became intrigued at the possibility of testing for the existence of the external answer bank.

I would like to now quote from a letter written to Karin about a test I devised to ascertain if an external answer bank existed.

Dear Karin,

I guess the time has come for me to test an idea in the book that you were kind enough to give me. Some of the ideas, as you said, sounded much like the material in my quiet thoughts notebook.

According to the author, individual man has a bank of answers that may be called upon within himself, and a bank of answers which exists outside him that also may be called upon.

I am going to test for the existence of this external answer bank in the same manner that I have used to confirm for myself the existence of a personal inner answer bank by asking that this question be answered: "How can people move freight practically by sound?"

If I get an answer to this question, as I usually do to my personal questions early in the morning, then I will have proven the existence of the bank of answers because I am not now aware of the answer, nor am I able to answer the question from my present life experience.

Sound was used, according to the author, by an earlier civilization to move things. If this is true, then quite possibly the principles involved were made a part of the external answer bank.

If my question goes unanswered, then this does not mean the answer bank does not exist; I realize an answer may be given in the form of a quiet thought which I do not recognize as the answer to my question. Or the answer may show up in my dreams, and I may not become aware of this quiet thought in my awake state. Or the answer may be given in terms that I do not understand. Or I may not be psychologically developed enough to receive the answer.

Well, let's see what unfolds. I thought that you might like to be in on this mind-expanding material from the start. Remember there are many failures before you strike one truth.

This is a most difficult undertaking because we are not just dealing with a state of mind, which is, in a manner of speaking, intangible. We are trying to prove the existence of an intangible answer bank as a result of achieving the tangible reality of moving freight by sound. We are also dealing here with the origin of ideas and quite possibly with a duplicatable process, which may be used by others to gain access to new ideas on a conscious level.

Love,
Tom

P.S. You know that I can't even remember your mailing address. How can I ever expect to learn to move freight by sound, when I can't even remember your address? Do you remember Ben Franklin, who flew a kite in a thunderstorm? I know I'm not Ben Franklin, but who knows what lies inside the human mind or soul unless someone tries? I reserve the right to call it off and chicken out. You see I'm scared — about the game I'm playing. And what does it mean for myself and others if I get an answer to my question?

Having set the stage to test for the existence of an external answer bank, I proceeded to ask this question before I went to sleep that night: "How do you practically move freight by sound?" In the morning I awoke with this quiet thought: *BECAUSE YOU ARE NOT CONVINCED OF THE NEED TO KNOW, THERE IS NO ANSWER.*

During the rest of that day I did not give much thought to how I was going to convince myself that I needed to know how to move freight practically by sound; instead, I tried to think up another question which, if answered, would prove to my satisfaction the existence of an external data bank. The question itself would have to satisfy two self-imposed requirements. One requirement was that the answer to the question had to be unknown in this civilization and, second, outside my present life experience.

That night I was still trying to figure out a question that would satisfy both requirements of being unknown and unanswerable from my experience. The latter requirement was easy to fulfill and could cover just about anything from Karin's address to astrology. But the first requirement, that I must personally be convinced of the need to know the answer to a question which was unknown to this civilization, was difficult. I was pondering this dilemma when I casually reached for a cigarette. I was reminded of my fear of getting lung cancer from smoking, and that was when

I hit upon this question: "What is a natural drug cure for cancer?"

This question fit my personal need-to-know requirement because if I ever contracted cancer, I could use the information on myself. And the question also fit my other requirement of being unknown to the present civilization. And as far as me being able to answer this question from my personal experience, that was impossible. For all intent and purposes, I was ignorant about the subject of cancer. I was pleased with my choice of question to help me test for the existence of an external answer bank.

Before I went to sleep that night, I asked myself this question: What is a natural drug cure for cancer? In the morning I awoke in the middle of a dream with an answer to my question, but I was too lazy to get out of bed to write down the quiet thought. I was violating one of my own rules about paying close attention to quiet thoughts, which, in this case, should have included immediately writing down the quiet thought at the time received. Later in the morning, when I finally got up, I forgot what the answer was to my question.

I thought there was no harm done because I would just re-ask the same question another night and in the morning I would be sure to write down the quiet thought promptly.

Before I even got an opportunity to re-ask the question, "What is a natural drug cure for cancer?" I lost all confidence in my abilities because I learned in my philosophical readings that night that god was not somehow responsible for me being able to provide answers. I was directly responsible for my successes in this area. When I realized this, I lost all confidence in my ability to learn answers to questions of this sort. As long as I thought that god was somehow responsible, then I was able to learn an answer. But without god's help I was unable to learn the answer. I did not even try that night to re-ask the question from the night before to which I knew I had received an answer.

Now instead of relying upon an explanation that god was somehow responsible for what I was able to do, I would have to use my own psychological and philosophical readings as a new foundation for explaining what I was able to do. No more would I be able to place the responsibility on god for what I was actually responsible for doing. I would have to accept total responsibility for both my successes and my failures. I realized it would take a period of time for me to adjust to my new way of thinking.

I really did not worry over this adjustment or my

new philosophy because I was busy preparing to leave for a trip abroad. I had been selected by the local Rotary District to join a study group in Denmark.

The Rotary Foundation of Rotary International, in conjunction with local clubs and districts, sponsors yearly group study exchange programs. I had earlier applied for this fellowship position and was now expected to join a group of young professional men who were to travel to Denmark.

While in Denmark, the group would be staying at the homes of local Rotarians to learn about their culture and to tell them something about the United States. On this trip, it would be a month before I met a person I felt comfortable enough with to talk openly about my psychic pursuits and interests.

This individual, whom I spent about a week with, enjoyed listening to my ideas. We exchanged views on many subjects. Because of his willingness to explore my new ideas, I brought him right up to date about my latest research project into learning about a cure for cancer. It was a blow-by-blow description, which left my host somewhat stunned about what I was trying to do. On the last night, I told him that I had regained my confidence enough to ask again for information on a cancer cure.

That night, before I went to sleep, I asked myself this question: What is the name of a natural drug cure for cancer and where is it found? In the morning I had this quiet thought, which I wrote down in three separate places so I would be sure not to lose track of the reply: *BARBIDOL, A SHRUB GROWN IN TEXAS.* Later in the day, I told my startled host I had learned about a cure, but I declined to mention the name. I wanted them to check and see if barbidol was the name of a shrub grown in Texas.

After I arrived home from Europe, I made a bee-line to the library to learn that my cure for cancer turned out to be non-existent. There was no such shrub grown in Texas, or anywhere else in the world, as far as I could tell. I shrugged off the experiment with a nothing-ventured, nothing-gained attitude.

I talked with Dave, a friend of mine, about this experiment, and he suggested that I check to see if there was a word in the dictionary close to "barbidol." We both checked further and decided the word "barbital" came closest in spelling to "barbidol." Barbital was a white crystalline powder used as a drug to induce sleep.

I made a mental note to do some further checking into barbital, but I wasn't excited. There was nothing in the word's definition to indicate the drug was a derivative of a shrub grown in Texas.

I was in no hurry to do further checking because, quite frankly, I didn't believe this quiet thought. I figured that unless the reply was one hundred percent accurate, I was not going any further. Little did I realize that psychics are not expected to be one hundred percent accurate all the time, especially on first attempts.

I was too busy during the next few months to be concerned about barbital, because I opened "The Center for Advanced Psychic Research and Development," which I hoped would enable me to teach people how to develop ESP abilities. It was enjoyable for me to find individuals who shared my interests in psychic phenomena. Several nights each week, I looked forward to sharing my ideas and philosophies about psychic phenomena. To prepare for each evening's class, I would usually spend the day reading books and articles on psychic phenomena.

I was up early on August 25, 1976. That morning was not unusual in any way. I had breakfast at about eight a.m. After breakfast, I went into the living room to do some more reading for the evening's ESP class. After a couple of hours, I decided to take a break.

During the break, I started to draft a letter to an organization in which I asked for specific information on barbital. First on my list of questions was: Is barbital a derivative of a shrub that grows in Texas? I was about half-way through the letter when Bob, another close friend, stopped by to say hello and generally pass the time of day.

After I told him what I was hoping to accomplish by writing this letter about barbital, he encouraged me to follow through on the cancer research project.

When Bob left, I decided I was wasting time by writing a letter; a phone call to the right party might bring quicker results. I called the State Agricultural Department and a research laboratory with no success. Then I made a call to a university library. The librarian told me that barbital was a manufactured drug. But she was unable to tell me if there was any connection between that drug and a shrub grown in Texas. I thanked her for the information and hung up. I was ready to give up on barbital and the whole cancer research project.

But, as I was walking from the kitchen into the living room, I had this quiet thought: *SUGGEST IN A DREAM STATE THAT MORE INFORMATION BE GIVEN, IDENTIFY EXACTLY, WHERE, HOW, AND*

WHEN. I almost dismissed this quiet thought, but I realized I had nothing to lose. I returned to the kitchen and made a note about this on the margin of the letter I had just drafted. I also said to myself in the margin note, that I had made this dream suggestion during the day when I was awake. This was a departure from my usual routine of making nighttime suggestions right before I went to sleep.

I returned to the living room and sat down to do more work in preparation for that evening's ESP class. During these classes, ESP phenomena were treated and explained as a natural outgrowth of human potential. No event was considered miraculous. I would explain the factors behind psychic phenomena to help members gain insight and/or develop the necessary mental framework which would then permit the experience of psychic phenomena. After an hour or so of reading, I got up and went into the bedroom to take a nap. I never even thought about making another specific dream suggestion, as I ordinarily would have done, because as soon as my head hit the pillow, I was fast asleep.

It appeared I had learned my lesson well about not writing down important quiet thoughts. As a direct result of my desire to learn of a natural drug for cancer and my desire not to forget the message or fail to write down the quiet thought, I was about to form a vivid dream I was not going to forget or ignore.

During this sleep, I was suddenly aware that I was wide awake in a dream in which I wrote by using light, a telepathic message as received in the same dream state. I wrote across what appeared to be a wide expanse the letters *"H-E-A-T-H-E-R."* I knew that whatever was being spelled out was a cure for cancer. I awoke, as startled as anyone might from any nightmare, to make sure I was all right. When I found myself okay, I went back to sleep again, just as I had done the first time that I had asked "What is a natural drug cure for cancer?" But this time, unlike the first, I was sure I would never forget those letters. When I finally awoke about half an hour later, I wrote down the word "heather."

The feelings or emotions I experienced after I had fully awakened are difficult to describe. The dreamer part of me did not want to return to this awake reality. I wanted to return to that state of mind of being fully awake in a dream.

Before I paint a picture so this psychic experience may be shared by the reader, I would like to point out the different stages of sleep which all of us experience.

Each night as we all turn away from our daily concerns, we enter the world of sleep. In the first stage of sleep, our inner senses make us alert to images and pictures. In the second stage we may become aware of voices and sounds. Then there comes a third stage in which telepathic messages may be received and understood, and light dreams may be formed. Finally, there is a fourth stage in which we are aware of the deepest reaches of our soul where we know pure knowing. As we awaken, there is a reversal of this process.

Most people usually remember only consciously the last two stages of their dreams, in which sounds or images are produced. Those of you who have already developed an ability to become awake in your dreams may be familiar with the other stages.

It was through telepathic messages received during the third stage of sleep that I was going to learn more about heather. Although I would usually only remember the telepathic message as a quiet thought and not as a vivid dream experience, the message itself was clear. But I did not know what heather was. The only connection in which I understood the word was as a girl's name. Not until I later looked up the word in the dictionary did I learn that heather was the name of an evergreen shrub. Then I made the immediate connection between the first message, "Barbidol, a shrub grown in Texas," and the second message, *"HEATHER,"* (an evergreen shrub). I was ecstatic and relieved over the connection. Five months had gone by since I first asked what is a natural drug cure for cancer.

The first matter I wanted to clear up was to understand the difference between the first message and the second message. In order to get this clarification, I suggested that night before I went to sleep that "I have a dream in which I receive a clarification between the first message, "Barbidol, a shrub grown in Texas" and the second message, *"HEATHER."* In the morning I had this quiet thought: *FIRST INACCURATE, SECOND ACCURATE.* I was pleased as punch with myself because these messages were finally intelligible. I was getting used to my own dreamer's shorthand in which quiet thoughts from external sources would now only make sense because of the questions that were asked. Without a knowledge of the question asked, the words, "first inaccurate, second accurate" would make no sense whatsoever.

The most important new ideas, which I accepted at the start of this research project, that allowed me to directly experience telepathic messages on a conscious level were 1) the conscious acceptance of the belief that answers could be learned from external sources and 2) learning of new ideas through telepathic means was not a mark of insanity. Without the conscious acceptance of the idea that learning of new ideas through telepathic means was a natural experience, I would never have permitted the conscious awareness of telepathic messages because I would have doubted my sanity. Were I to have asked the question concerning cancer while still believing I could learn the information using traditional methodologies, another more ordinary means might have been arranged to learn the answer. I was prepared to handle telepathic messages as the direct result of years of training in dealing with quiet thoughts from my own inner sources. Another person might not need years of training to experience mental telepathy on a conscious level but might simply accept telepathy as the natural experience, which it is.

Quiet thoughts did sometimes have a way of conflicting with beliefs. In this instance, for example, I became confused over exactly what was supposed to be cured cancer or leukemia. I put this question aside momentarily and went to the library to find out what

I could about heather.

When I got to the library, I learned from a book that the heather grew in many parts of the world. I also remember mispronouncing the word "heather" as health'er instead of using the correct pronunciation, heth'er. At the same moment, I experienced this quick quiet thought, which was not based on anything in the book: *THE PLANT WAS USED IN THE 15TH CENTURY AS A MEDICINAL HERB AND FOR QUITE SOME TIME BEFORE. BUT MAN HAD SINCE FORGOTTEN THE HEALTH USES TO WHICH THE DRUG WAS PUT.*

It then dawned on me that my imagination might be playing tricks and this experience might be the product of some wishful thinking. I experienced the same doubts any person might feel when he realizes he is directly experiencing telepathic messages. These same doubts were soon to be calmed, however. As you will remember, I selected the question "What is a natural drug cure for cancer?" because it was not within my present life experience to know the answer and also because I was, for all intents and purposes, ignorant about the subject of cancer. My ignorance about the subject was soon to be pointed out, but my fears that my imagination was running away from me calmed at the same time, as a result of receiving an answer to the following question. I asked this question: Which disease does heather cure, cancer or leukemia? Most readers, I am sure, will recognize immediately that leukemia is a form of cancer. I did not realize this when I asked the question. You can imagine my amazement in the morning when I had this quiet thought, *"BOTH."*

Now I was even more confused than ever, heather was supposed to cure both diseases, cancer and leukemia. I thought to myself, how can that be, when they are two different diseases, and especially when I only asked what is a natural drug for cancer, not leukemia? It was not until later in the day that I learned leukemia was a form of cancer. As a matter of fact, I was glad leukemia was a form of cancer. The fact that I was glad leukemia was a form of cancer is not in any way to be construed to mean that I take anything I am saying here lightly. I approached what I was trying to do now with the utmost seriousness and secrecy. The humor and game-like attitude with which I approached my psychic pursuits was gone when it came time to deal with this project of discovering a cure for cancer. I was looking for any sign, projection or quiet thought that might indicate my imagination was running away with itself. I was ready to drop the entire project at any time I felt that what I was doing was wrong or the information received was incorrect. The quiet thought *BOTH* relieved the tension. At least, I thought to myself, if my imagination was playing tricks on me I would have selected one or the other, because consciously I thought the two diseases were different.

I did not want to take a chance that the connection I had developed with my telepathic partner would be lost. I had once before lost the connection when I lost all confidence in my abilities to obtain answers to questions, so I continued asking questions. I attempted to ask as many questions as I could about cancer treatment before I tried to learn about the source of these replies. Conscious awareness of mental telepathy of this type is a difficult state of mind to maintain in the early stages of development. Many factors can upset the psychological preparation required to achieve this open channel.

Briefly, for those readers who are not familiar with mental telepathy, I would like to state what occurs between the sender and the receiver of thought waves. When a person thinks a thought, he produces two sets of thought waves. One set is internalized for inner use, and the other set is sent out, which the receiver duplicates with his own thought wave. This new wave is then internalized by the receiver for his own use.

Before my afternoon nap, I asked this question: What part of the plant is used? *ROOTS, CUT ONE INCH BELOW THE STEM, GROUND, ADD HOT BOILING WATER* was the reply.

I tried to think up things that I thought would be important to ask about this drug treatment. I tried to ask simple direct questions. What is the potency and the effect of the drugs? *WEAK TO STRONG, MOLECULAR STRUCTURE OF THE CELLS RESTORED.*

I never had to worry that I was having a hallucination because of some drug I was using because at the time I used no drugs whatsoever, even when I was sick. I was reminded of my first quiet thoughts about finding a drug cure for cancer by using animals, in which I said, *BUT IT* (the drug) *WILL SERVE THOSE WHO, BECAUSE OF THEIR BELIEFS, SEE DRUGS AS THE CURE. THE NATURAL CURE RESTS OUTSIDE THE CAGES AND BUILDINGS THAT SERVE TO CONTAIN OUR CONSCIOUS KNOWLEDGE AND RESTRAIN THE ANIMALS FROM SHOWING US THE WAY.*

REMEMBER PENICILLIN? It was at this point that I drew an analogy between heather and penicillin. I now understood, too, why I had also written down, sometime back, *THE KNOWLEDGE THAT YOU SEEK IS ALREADY AVAILABLE TO US.* It appeared that the person with whom I was now in contact was then working behind the scenes to help prepare me to receive, through conscious awareness of mental telepathy, this new information.

I did hold some preconceived ideas about cancer as the result of some newspaper articles and a passage in a book that I had read which briefly considered the possible causes of cancer. I say this now because any telepathic message a person might become aware of is colored by the receiver's attitudes, just as what you read here is colored by your own attitudes and experiences. For this and other reasons, I know the material I am now presenting is meant to serve only as a general guideline. When I asked the person with whom I was in telepathic communication what the cause of cancer was, this was the response: *VIRUS ALREADY PRESENT WITHIN THE CELLS ARE ACTED UPON BY THE MIND SO THAT EXCRETIONS ARE PRODUCED WHICH CAUSE A CHEMICAL IMBALANCE WITHIN THE CELLS.*

At another time, I asked if the disease could be produced by means other than the virus and the mind. *YES, THE CHEMICAL IMBALANCE MAY BE ARTIFICIALLY PRODUCED BY BY-PASSING THE VIRUS BUT THERE MUST BE AN ACCEPTANCE OF THE DISEASE BY THE INDIVIDUAL. THE INDIVIDUAL PERMITS THE PHYSICAL EXPERIENCE OF THIS DISEASE AND EVERY DISEASE FOR THEIR OWN PERSONAL REASONS.*

I wondered about what I should do with the information I had thus far learned. So, I asked before I went to sleep, what am I to do next? *NOTHING, NO ONE IS GOING TO BELIEVE YOU.* I decided to not follow this quiet thought. Instead, I wrote to several organizations offering them the information I had thus far received. I wanted to have the material tested, so I could find out if the material I identified was right or wrong. I also did not want to continue with the psychic research project if the data received was incorrect.

I first wrote to pharmaceutical firms who were very interested in learning about a drug to cure cancer. But when I wrote to them proposing a natural drug as a treatment, these same firms were no longer interested. They were only interested in a substance which could be synthesized for sale to the public.

I was intensely eager to let others (besides my close, immediate friends, who agreed not to tell anyone about the drug until it was successfully tested) know what I had learned. I wanted to share the story about my experiences and have the data tested. I decided one day to tell my ESP class of my psychic adventure but without telling the name of the drug. After I related the story, one of the students suggested I write a particular organization in New York which was noted for its cancer research. I thanked the student for her advice and said I would conduct a future probability test on contacting that organization.

In this instance, a future probability test boils down to learning what would happen *if* this organization in New York tested heather in the manner prescribed. I asked this question before I went to sleep that same night: What will the results be if the New York organization tests heather on humans as prescribed? Early in the morning came this quiet thought: *FINDINGS CONFIRMED*.

Elated at the early prospects of having my findings confirmed, I immediately wrote a letter to the New York organization offering them the information I had received in return for a signed agreement acknowledging the fact that I supplied the original data.

I then returned to asking questions about the nature of the drug itself and related questions. When my natural curiosity did not prompt good, consciously-directed questions, I later learned my telepathic partner was working behind the scenes again to make sure that I asked the right questions by suggesting the questions to be asked. I also learned that I willingly approved of this arrangement in a dream state. On a conscious level, my desire for answers gave tacit approval of this arrangement. Why was it, I wondered, necessary to make a one-inch cut below the stem? *THIS PERMITS THE SHRUB TO BE REPLANTED AND USED AGAIN IN TWO YEARS*, I was told. "I never would have thought of that explanation on my own," I thought to myself.

Because I wanted to minimize any possible distractions in receiving objective answers, I usually used my sleep state to receive answers to questions. Here, I thought the distractions would be minimized and there would be little chance of other ideas coming into play. I felt the nature of the material dictated that I use extreme care. It would be up to others to alter, change, or interpret the data as a result of their own tests on heather. I was not in a position to test the data myself.

I asked several questions, over three or four days, to prompt these quiet thoughts (which still came in the form of unspoken words, phrases, or sentences) regarding drug preparation. *WATER IS USED TO WASH THE PLANTS OF ALL FOREIGN MATTER. THEN THE ROOTS ARE CUT ONE INCH BELOW THE STEMS. THE REMAINING ROOTS ARE DRIED AND CURED IN NATURAL SUNLIGHT WHICH IS BEST FOR CURING PURPOSES. THEN THE THOROUGHLY DRIED AND CURED ROOTS ARE GROUND. DO NOT FORGET TO SOON REPLANT THE SHRUB FOR LATER USE.*

Because I thought the New York organization might want to have a sample of the drug, I asked questions about storage and handling. *THE DRUG IN ITS NATURAL DRY STATE REQUIRES NO SPECIAL HANDLING. HOWEVER, NORMAL REFRIGERATION WILL RETARD DECOMPOSITION.*

I finally asked whom I was obtaining this information from one night before I went to sleep. I learned the person wished at this time to be identified only as a *"DOCTOR."*

I am now going to combine and edit certain replies to my questions which were extended over a year and a half to facilitate an orderly presentation of the data learned through telepathic communications.

When I asked the doctor what dosages were to be given, this was the quiet thought: *ONE TO TWO OUNCES, DEPENDING UPON THE POTENCY EXPECTED, ARE ADDED TO HOT WATER AND TAKEN DAILY. THE ENTIRE DOSAGE OF ONE OR TWO OUNCES SHOULD BE ADMINISTERED IN TWO OR THREE SEPARATE DOSAGES DURING THE DAY. NORMAL SLEEP PATTERNS ARE NOT TO BE BROKEN TO ADMINISTER THE DRUG. NO OTHER MEDICATIONS ARE TO BE GIVEN DURING THE TIME THIS DRUG IS ADMINISTERED BECAUSE OF POSSIBLE ADVERSE REACTIONS FROM USING THE OTHER DRUG AT THE SAME TIME. THE BODY IS CAPABLE OF HANDLING THE ROOT OF THE HEATHER SHRUB IF GIVEN IN THE DRUG'S NATURAL STATE. CAUTION: THIS IS A DRUG AND IS NOT A FOOD IN THE GENERALLY ACCEPTED MEANING OF THE WORD "FOOD." IT IS NOT TO BE USED FOR NON-MEDICAL PURPOSES.*

I later learned that in some localities heather is called heath, which is known to have toxic strains. The botanical designation of heather is *Calluna Vulgaris*

[L.]. Caution is advised in selecting the correct plant and strain.

I was puzzled about why you add hot or boiling water, so I asked for an explanation. *THE HOT WATER, WHICH AIDS DIGESTION, SHOULD BE COOL ENOUGH AT THE TIME OF INGESTION TO PERMIT SWALLOWING.* Later I learned it was the intention of the doctor that the *INFORMATION PROVIDED SHOULD BE UTILIZED AND UNDERSTOOD BY THE LAYMAN WHO IS NOT BOUND BY THE RULES AND REGULATIONS OF SOCIETY WHICH MAY PROHIBIT THE USE OF UNAPPROVED DRUGS.*

I was still trying to get the data tested by scientific organizations and experts in the field of cancer, who I thought would provide an objective decision about the merits of heather. I sent out letters to twenty-five organizations that received grants for cancer research. I hoped one would become interested in testing the information. I agreed to provide them with the data in return for a signed agreement stating I provided them with the original information on heather. Some organizations responded but most simply did not reply. A few of the respondents directed me to a national research organization to which I immediately wrote.

Then I heard from the New York organization which was interested in testing heather.

My excitement over receiving a letter from the New York organization (and later a secrecy agreement which I signed) to test my proposed cure was short-lived. After I provided them with the information, I was asked to supply them with animal tumor-testing data, which I was not in a position to provide. They assumed my cancer cure was already tested on animals. In later correspondence, I was told this organization would first have to check with the same national research organization that I had just written, to see if tests had been conducted there on heather before conducting their own tests.

I decided to test for future probabilities again to ascertain for myself what exactly would happen as a result of my efforts to get heather tested. This was not the same as the future probability test in which I proposed to find out what would happen if tests of the material were conducted on humans as prescribed by the doctor. I was only successful once in getting replies to my questions. When I asked what would happen at one organization in response to a letter I was planning to send about the drug, this was the quiet thought: *THE LETTER WOULD BE LAUGHED AT.* Not wanting to be laughed at, I recomposed the letter. But when I asked again, there was no response. In serious matters like this, when I asked about future probabilities, I had come to expect replies. It was very unusual not to get a reply. When I re-asked the question, there was still no response. There was no quiet thought. Once you become used to knowing beforehand what is going to happen, you learn to depend on these insights to determine what you should do or not do. But in this instance, and regarding these questions, I was in the dark about what was going to happen.

Once in a while, I would establish direct dream-state telepathic communication with the person at the organization I was dealing with to find out what was going on. When I asked, for example, the person in the New York organization, in a dream, what was going on, I awoke in the middle of the night to find out *NOTHING WAS BEING DONE.* The next week, to confirm this quiet thought, I wrote a letter asking about the current status. I was told, again, that an inquiry had not yet been made to the national testing organization. Later, I learned that it was because my questions would have brought negative replies that I did not learn what was going to happen. If I knew consciously what was going to happen beforehand, I would have stopped all efforts to get these organizations to test my material.

I continued the nightly task of asking questions before I went to sleep in the hopes that I would soon hear from the national research organization, which appeared to be my last hope of finding out about the correctness of the material. Here are some of the replies that I learned. *THE DRUG SHOULD NOT BE COOKED, BAKED OR FROZEN TO INSURE THAT DRUG POTENCY IS NOT INJURED, ALTHOUGH THE DRUG MAY BE ADDED TO OTHER FOOD STUFFS SERVED AT ROOM TEMPERATURE TO SUIT INDIVIDUAL TASTE PREFERENCES. INGESTION OF THE DRUG IN THE RAW STATE INSURES THAT THE REQUIRED CHEMICAL ACTIONS AND REACTIONS TAKE PLACE WITHIN THE BODY.*

I became concerned about how long a person should take the drug. This led to this response: *THE DRUG IS TAKEN ORALLY UNTIL THE CONDITION IS ARRESTED, WHICH IS USUALLY TWO WEEKS TO A MONTH.* Without prompting or asking about when to discontinue the treatment, I learned: *DISCONTINUE THIS TREATMENT IF THERE IS NO*

HEALING IN TWO MONTHS.

I became interested in the effectiveness of heather, so I asked what may be expected. The doctor replied, *SEVENTY PERCENT OF ALL TREATED CASES.* Then, for some inexplicable reason, I put down a lower percentage figure of expected effectiveness. My actions were to be understood in the light of what I later learned. The lower figure was correct when I wrongly assumed heather could cure all forms of cancer. The higher figure of seventy percent was more correct because the doctor did not intend or state that all forms of cancer would be cured by heather. The doctor said *CERVICAL AND BREAST CANCER, LEUKEMIA AND CERTAIN FORMS OF SKIN CANCER WOULD BE CURED. LUNG CANCER, FOR EXAMPLE, WOULD REQUIRE A DIFFERENT DRUG.*

When I first started receiving messages on cancer, I decided it might be a good idea if I stayed away from literature on cancer. I wanted to remain as objective as possible. When I asked what diseases heather was supposed to treat, the reply was only leukemia and certain other forms of cancer including skin, cervical, and breast cancer; I was puzzled over the word "cervical" because I did not know what the word meant. When I looked cervical up in the small dictionary, I found the word pertained to the neck region and to any cervix. Because I never heard of cancer of the neck, I debated over whether I should include this in my report. I finally decided I would put down the message as received. I justified my reason for including this term because I believed my doctor friend might know something that I didn't. I felt that possibly a subsequent reader of the report might take action on the information because he had a friend who had cancer of the neck region. I thought this was the doctor's reason for wanting the information included in a report which I later sent to an organization for testing. I never did ask the doctor directly why he wished me to include cervical in with the diseases to be cured.

Another friend of mine, Ron, tried to keep me abreast of any news dealing with cancer. One night he called and asked if I had read about a new drug treatment. I thought for a minute that another person might have hit upon the idea of using heather and that I was wasting my time trying to get something tested that was already in use. I said, "No, I haven't seen anything about a new drug treatment, what's the name of the drug?" Ron responded, "Laetrile." I then told

Ron I would first ask my source of information about laetrile and then I would try to get the article. Although I did not read about laetrile in that newspaper, I asked my doctor friend what his opinion was: *THE DIRECT MEDICAL VALUE OF LAETRILE AS A THERAPEUTIC DRUG IS DOUBTFUL, APART FROM THE PSYCHOLOGICAL VALUE WHICH MAY BE OF SOME CONSEQUENCE.* It wasn't until three months later, when I read an article in a magazine about laetrile which seemed to confirm the doctor's opinion, that I felt absolutely certain I had in fact learned a cancer cure. It was not because the doctor's opinion on laetrile was confirmed, but because I learned there was a disease called cervical cancer. I was elated over this discovery, more than anything else I had learned to date, because three months earlier I had included cervical cancer as one of the conditions that would be cured by heather, without knowing what the word meant. This signaled that I was being as objective as possible in relaying the information received to interested persons.

When I asked one of the girls at work what cervical cancer was, I was told that cervical cancer is a female disease that attacks the cervix part of the womb. I was embarrassed over my lack of knowledge of certain female parts of the body. As you can see, learning and insights into the nature of cancer do not make me a final authority on cancer.

My anxiousness over what would happen when heather was finally used by a patient prompted me to take a peek into the flexible future. Without the doctor's help, I conducted a future probability test by asking this question. Please note that the question was "What will the effect be on the first patient who uses this natural drug as directed?" My quiet thought on this matter also included the effects on the second and third patients as well. Had I stopped with the first patient, I might have put a stop to this psychic research project altogether. This is the quiet thought which was learned while I was fully awake: *THE FIRST PERSON TO RECEIVE THE DRUG DOES NOT OVERCOME THE DISEASE BECAUSE OF A STRONG BELIEF IN THE ILLNESS AND A LACK OF BELIEF IN THE POWER OF THE DRUG, IN THE SELF, AND IN THE DOCTOR TO CURE THE ILLNESS. THE SECOND AND THIRD DO RECOVER WITHIN ONE OR TWO WEEKS AS A RESULT OF THEIR BELIEF IN THE POWER OF DRUGS AND THE DOCTORS, AS PREDICTED. THE FIRST PERSON UPON HEARING OF THE RESULTS ACHIEVED BY THE OTHER TWO*

PERSONS HAS A MIRACULOUS HEALING. THIS IS NOT THE EFFECT OF THE DRUG TREATMENTS WHICH HAVE BEEN DISCONTINUED BUT AS A RESULT OF THE BELIEFS OF THE INDIVIDUAL THAT HAVE BEEN ALTERED. THE BELIEFS OF THE PERSON TO CURE HIMSELF HAVE BEEN STRENGTHENED BY THE ACTIONS AND THE RESULTS ACHIEVED BY THE OTHER TWO PATIENTS. THIS WILL SERVE TO ILLUSTRATE THE POWER OF AN INDIVIDUAL TO CURE HIMSELF BY USING THE RESOURCES OF HIS MIND THROUGH HIS CONSCIOUS BELIEFS. IT WILL BE REGARDED AS A DELAYED REACTION ON THE PART OF THE DRUG AND THIS PRONOUNCEMENT WILL MAKE THE DRUG EVEN MORE EFFECTIVE THAN ORIGINALLY THOUGHT.

As I was shifting my focus away from this exact point in time, I tried to refocus my attention back to when this was supposed to happen. I was seeking an exact date, but the date obtained is wrong by our time standards. The flexible nature of time and why this date is wrong by our time standards is better left, ironically, to another point in time to explain. Also, I would like to be better able to give the reader practical illustrations from further research into the nature of time and events. My doctor friend does not care to comment because of the difficulties involved in giving specific dates. He knows better than to give specific dates because of the flexible nature of time and events.

After I had done this psychic future probability study which held all sorts of promise that heather would ultimately be found effective, I learned from the New York organization that heather had been extensively tested with negative results at the national research organization. Then I learned directly from the national research organization that although their tests were negative, they would be willing to test my data. I was not glad to hear heather had already been tested with negative results, but I was glad that at least someone else before me had suggested heather as a cure for cancer. As far as I was concerned, this was my last attempt to have the data tested. If their results proved negative, then I was finished with the project and with trying to prove the existence of an external answer bank. My only comment regarding the negative results, in a report I later sent them, was that "More information regarding their testing procedures would have to be supplied." I believed the only way I could ask the doctor his opinion on the testing procedures was to have this information in front of me. But later events would point out that the doctor was way ahead of me.

I decided I would try to make this report that I would send the national organization as complete as possible. To achieve this, I continued asking more questions.

Questions regarding plant selection and growth brought these replies or quiet thoughts: *EARLY FALL OR LATE SPRING HARVESTING IS BEST. SOIL TESTS MAY BE CONDUCTED TO DETERMINE THE DEGREE OF AMMONIUM NITRATE IN THE SOIL. HIGH LEVELS OF AMMONIUM NITRATE WILL TEND TO INDICATE STRONG DRUG POTENCY. PLANTS GROWN IN A NURSERY WILL PERFORM BETTER THAN THOSE GROWN IN THE WILD. PLANTS ULTIMATELY SELECTED FROM BOTANICAL GARDENS RAISED BY GROWERS WITH THE MENTAL EXPECTATION THAT THESE SAME PLANTS WILL ACHIEVE A HIGH DEGREE OF DRUG POTENCY WILL ACHIEVE A HIGHER DEGREE OF DRUG POTENCY AS A RESULT OF THE DIRECT MENTAL INTERACTIONS BETWEEN PLANTS AND GROWERS.*

As to questions to the doctor regarding drug potency, this is the doctor's opinion: *THE POTENCY*

VARIES FROM WEAK TO STRONG DEPENDING UPON THE CLIMATE, GROWING CONDITION, AND THE AMOUNT OF AMMONIUM NITRATE IN THE SOIL. THE STRONGEST MEDICAL PROPERTIES ARE LOCATED IN THE ROOTS.

I am going to preface the doctor's remarks on patient attitude with some remarks of my own in the hope that any adverse views a person may hold about drugs, doctors, and self to cure an illness will be overcome. It should come as no surprise to anyone that, without a person's willing consent, no drug will be effective. It is possible to cure a disease through a non-therapeutic agent such as a sugar tablet. Likewise, it is possible for a person to block, for his own reasons, the medicinal effect of drugs and drug treatment. In order to remedy this situation, attention must be focused away for a time from these less than helpful views to a view that is more beneficial, thereby allowing a drug to work properly in his body. By dwelling upon this new direction for no more than ten minutes daily, beginning two weeks before and during the entire length of time the drug is administered, most persons will react better to a drug treatment: "I direct all my adverse ideas I hold about drugs, doctors, and myself to cure this illness were a part of my personality. I direct myself to no longer hold these old ideas. Now, in this new moment, I willingly accept the new view I want that this drug will return me to good health."

These are the doctor's comments on patient attitude: *APART FROM INDIVIDUAL BODY CHEM-ISTRIES, A PATIENT WITH A STRONG BELIEF IN THE POWER OF DRUGS AND DOCTORS WITH A WILL TO LIVE IN PHYSICAL REALITY AND SOMETHING TO LIVE FOR WILL REACT BETTER TO THE DRUG. THE PERSON SHOULD NOT BE IN THE THROES OF DEATH AND THIS DRUG GIVEN AS A LAST RESORT IN THE INITIAL TESTING OF THE SUBSTANCE.*

I did not always become aware of telepathic messages from the doctor as soon as I awoke in the morning or by becoming awake in a dream. Sometimes these messages became a part of memory, which I would recall when needed in the form of a direct quiet thought or in a projected quiet thought. For example, when I asked about human effectiveness expected, I got this answer: "seventy percent of treated cases." Later I would become aware of why this drug will not cure all persons, although no direct question was ever asked. *THIS DRUG WILL NOT CURE ALL TREATED*

CASES BECAUSE OF MANY FACTORS INCLUDING INDIVIDUAL BODY CHEMISTRIES, TYPE OF ILL-NESS, PATIENT ATTITUDE, STAGE OF ILLNESS, AND PLANT POTENCY, AMONG OTHERS.

Inquiries regarding animal effectiveness for the report to the national research organization brought this response: *THIS DRUG WORKS BETTER IN HUMANS AND IS ONLY SLIGHTLY EFFECTIVE IN ANIMALS BECAUSE OF THE DIFFERENT CHEMISTRIES INVOLVED.*

Quiet thoughts on any possible side effects included the following: *IN THE NATURAL DRY STATE, HEATHER, TAKEN IN NORMAL AMOUNTS, IS READILY ACCEPTED BY THE BODY AS FOOD AND BADLY NEEDED NOURISHMENT. IT IS NON-TOXIC AND NO ADVERSE SIDE EFFECTS ARE EXPECTED WHEN USED IN THE PROPER DOSAGES AS RECOMMENDED. AGAIN, CAUTION IS ADVISED BECAUSE THIS IS A DRUG AND NOT A FOOD IN THE GENERALLY ACCEPTED MEANING OF THE WORD "FOOD."*

The material on effects of the drug within the cells was the most difficult information to obtain because of my lack of biological expertise. Over and over again, I had to re-state the same questions, trying to make sense out of quiet thoughts that used words and terms I was not familiar with. I felt persons at the national research center would be most interested in this data and would be better able to interpret or understand what follows. *THE MOLECULAR STRUCTURE OF THE CELLS IS RESTORED BY PROVIDING THE NECESSARY NUTRIENTS AND PROTEINS FOR THE BODY TO CORRECT THE CHEMICAL IMBALANCE WITHIN THE CELLS CAUSED BY THE PARTICULAR STRAIN OF VIRUS INVOLVED IN MOST CASES. THE DNA MOLECULES ARE AFFECTED IN A POSITIVE WAY TO CORRECT THE CHEMICAL IMBALANCES.*

IN THIS INSTANCE, PROTEINS ACT AS THE AGENT FOR CHANGE. ENZYMES HAVE A STRONG RESISTANCE TO CHANGE THAT MUST BE OVERCOME BY AN OUTSIDE AGENT. THE AGENT IN THIS CASE IS THE DRUG.

THE START OF THE SECOND WEEK OF TREATMENT IS CRITICAL BECAUSE ENZYME RESISTANCE TO CHANGE IS STRONG AND MUST BE OVERCOME. AN OLD ENZYME STRUCTURE IS BEING TORN DOWN AND A NEW ENZYME STRUCTURE IS BEING BUILT. THE ENZYMES SEEK TO RETAIN THEIR OLD IDENTITY AND

STRUCTURE.

A CHEMICAL ACTION AND REACTION TAKES PLACE WITHIN THE CELL IN WHICH THE DRUG PROVIDES BOTH THE CATALYST FOR THE BREAKDOWN AND THE NECESSARY NUTRIENTS FOR THE NEW STRUCTURE. CERTAIN NUTRIENTS AND PROTEINS CURRENTLY LACKING IN THE BODY IN SUFFICIENT NUMBER, PRODUCTION OR PROPORTION ARE PROVIDED FOR BY THE DRUG.

AT THE START OF THE SECOND WEEK OF TREATMENT, THE BREAKDOWN PROCESS IS COMPLETED AND THE NEW STRUCTURE BEGUN. THROUGH THE NATURAL NUTRIENT SELECTION PROCESS, THE INDIVIDUAL MAKES THE CALCULATIONS TO DETERMINE THE EXACT PROPORTION OF TWO DIFFERENT COMPOUNDS TO BE ACCEPTED AND USED BY THE BODY. THE PROPORTIONS OF THE TWO COMPOUNDS WILL VARY DURING THE DIFFERENT STAGES OF THE TREATMENT AS THE ILLNESS IS BEING OVERCOME.

AFTER THE EFFECTIVENESS OF THE DRUG IS DEMONSTRATED IN THE NATURAL STATE, EXACT IDENTIFICATION OF THE TWO ACTIVE INGREDIENTS MAY BE MADE. IN THE PRESENT

NATURAL STATE, THE DRUG IS SAFE AND EFFECTIVE.

On the advice of the doctor, I made no attempt to identify the two compounds within the root of heather because such identification is not needed at this time. I also learned *THERE DO EXIST OTHER NATURAL DRUGS AND SOME PREPARED REMEDIES WHICH WILL TREAT **ALL** FORMS OF CANCER.*

I compiled the information I had thus far received from the doctor into an abstract, and sent it on to the national research center. I also sent other information regarding cancer treatment that I thought would be useful for testing and evaluation. I thought at the very least the report would provide a general framework for other scientists to work from. It was not expected to be 100 percent accurate, but I thought the data had merit and should be tested.

I thought I finally had succeeded in finding an organization that was willing to test my material as prescribed. After a year and a half of writing letters to organizations inviting them to test the material, the finding of just one organization which was willing to test the material was a rewarding feeling.

I had started my first series of letters to pharmaceutical firms. These firms were only interested in manufactured chemical substances and not in natural drugs. My letters to national foundations brought no replies. My phone calls and personal visits to cancer foundations brought no results. My inquiries to publicly-supported centers for cancer research brought a few responses that directed me to this national research organization, the one I had just sent a report. As far as I was concerned, this national cancer research center was the end of the road. I thought back to the time I first asked the doctor what I should do next and the reply was: *NOTHING, NO ONE IS GOING TO BELIEVE YOU.*

It was not long before I got back a letter from the national research center. In the letter was a request that I submit a sample of the drug that I wished to have tested.

I went to a nursery the next day to purchase the four or five shrubs of heather I thought would be sufficient for testing. The owner of the nursery asked me to return during normal working hours the next day to pick up the shrubs which he would dig up for me early in the morning.

I thought it would be interesting to learn beforehand what the results would be using future probability tests on the results that would be obtained by the national cancer research organization. This is, as you will recall, a psychic procedure that may be used beforehand to determine what will happen as a result of taking a particular course of action. That night, just before I went to sleep, I asked this question: "What will the results be at the national cancer research center of the heather?" I was stunned by the early morning quiet thought that brought this answer to that question: *THE RESULTS OF THE TEST WILL BE NEGATIVE. . . . . BECAUSE THE HUMAN FACTOR IS NOT INVOLVED.*

The language I used and the expletives can be best described as total disgust over what I had just learned. I was shaken by this quiet thought. I thought about the many hours of work that had gone into this project, gathering information on a drug that would not be proven effective at the national cancer research center. I immediately wrote a letter to the center about what I had just learned. I asked them to update my report with this new finding. *IT WAS LEARNED TODAY THAT THE RESULTS FROM YOUR TESTING CONDITIONS WOULD BE NEGATIVE BECAUSE "THE HUMAN FACTOR IS NOT INVOLVED." IT WAS BECAUSE OF THIS FINDING AND THE IMPLICATIONS WHICH YOUR TEST RESULTS*

WOULD HAVE FOR OTHERS THAT I HAVE DECIDED NOT TO SEND A SAMPLE OF HEATHER ROOT.

The decision not to send a sample of heather consisting of several roots was easy to make. There was no reason for me to question the quiet thought because it was very distinct and clear. No further questions were raised in my mind over this quiet thought. It was the opposite reply I had hoped for when I asked the question about what the results would be.

I was now thinking on a selfish level. What implications did this have for me? I had hoped the national cancer research organization would test the material themselves directly on humans. It was not long before I learned from the center that they were prohibited from directly testing drugs on humans. When I learned that tests would not be conducted on humans directly but would be done on animals, I felt lost. Because I was not a doctor, I didn't feel I could administer the drug to any patient. I thought I would never learn if I was right or wrong about my cancer findings. Nor would I be able to prove if I had tapped into some external answer bank which originally led me to ask about a natural drug cure for cancer.

The logic behind over a year and a half of inviting people to test the material as prescribed evaded me. It seemed I had gone a long way for nothing. It was difficult for a person who has grown accustomed to asking himself questions regarding personal problems to not ask himself what the solution was to this particular dilemma, and why this particular course of action, which now seemed so futile, was selected over other possible alternatives that might have had more positive results. So, shortly after I received the letter from the national organization telling me no direct human tests could be conducted, I asked myself why this course of action was taken.

This was the quiet thought: *THIS STEP OF OFFERING THE INFORMATION TO THESE ORGANIZATIONS WAS NECESSARY BEFORE PUBLICATION OF THESE FINDINGS WITHOUT TESTING WAS JUSTIFIED.*

If I had known in the beginning that no organization was going to test the material exactly as prescribed from the start, I never would have vigorously pursued that task of trying to get the material tested. *BEFORE YOU BEGIN WORK ON A BOOK, YOU SHOULD BEGIN GATHERING INFORMATION ON IMMUNIZATION FROM ALL*

FORMS OF CANCER.
"My god," I thought to myself, "who is ever going to believe me now?"

Chapter Four
ON IMMUNIZATION

My way of learning about immunization through telepathic communications with the doctor did involve some procedural changes. Instead of asking questions for information on immunization against cancer, I allowed him to relay or communicate any information that he considered important. I would then recall the sometimes lengthy quiet thoughts. Now I would only ask questions when I thought the material was unclear or when I thought a question was proper. I am sure, as I continue to experience mental telepathy from the doctor or from other sources, there may be some other procedural changes.

Because the doctor had recommended the use of a natural substance to cure certain types of cancers, I thought I would learn the formula for a serum which would immunize people against cancer. I had the preconceived idea that he would at least give some admonitions against smoking cigarettes. One only had to listen to news broadcasters to learn about this drug or that chemical which was proved to be a cancer causing agent. I thought there would also be some news about staying away from this chemical or even a certain manufactured product. I was open to any type of suggestion he was ready to make. It was a good thing I had opened myself up to receive whatever his opinion was because what I expected to learn and what I learned turned out to be two different things.

The doctor expected interested persons to act upon his prescription for immunization as they would for their own personal physician. Without this, no prescription would help, and they would be no better off tomorrow than they were today in protecting themselves from cancer. Without this action on the individual's part, the doctor feared cancer would grow to epidemic proportions. He placed responsibility for any epidemic on well-intentioned but misguided individuals who did not realize what their scare tactics were ultimately doing when they broadcast news about the possible causes of cancer. The doctor thinks his timely action would head off a dangerous condition now being created by mankind. He states that the best line of defense against cancer rests with the individual. The doctor says the information provided may be used to immunize a person from any disease in addition to cancer. In this way, he thought his actions were not only timely but timeless, as these procedures may also be used by future generations to effect immunity against other diseases.

I learned of four separate immunization alternatives that a person may use to keep his body free of all forms of cancer. I also learned of two other immunity alternatives that could be used to immunize other persons unable to effect immunity themselves by using the first four alternatives. All of the alternatives may be compared to the many branches of a single tree. Each branch is different, but all branches together make up the tree of immunity. The type of immunity the doctor talks about is effective mental immunization against a particular disease.

The doctor, through my quiet thoughts, now speaks on IMMUNIZATION: *AN INDIVIDUAL MAY USE A FACULTY OF HIS MIND TO PRODUCE CERTAIN ANTIBODIES AGAINST A PARTICULAR DISEASE. THIS STATE OF BODY MAY BE BROUGHT ABOUT THROUGH THE*

CONSTRUCTION OF A CERTAIN BELIEF SYSTEM. THE NEW BELIEF SYSTEM MAY BE BROUGHT ABOUT IN A MANNER I WILL DESCRIBE WITH THE AUTHOR'S HELP. IT IS NOT DIFFICULT. IT IS EASY.

THE FIRST STEP IN BRINGING ABOUT IMMUNIZATION FROM ALL FORMS OF CANCER THROUGH MENTAL PROCESSES IS THE CONSIDERATION BY THE INDIVIDUAL OF HIS OWN BELIEFS. WITHOUT TRUE REGARD FOR HIS OWN BELIEFS BY THE INDIVIDUAL, ANY IMMUNIZATION TECHNIQUES PROPOSED MIGHT BE SHORT-CIRCUITED. IT DOES NOT MATTER WHAT YOUR CURRENT BELIEFS ARE. IT IS UNDERSTOOD BY ME THAT MOST OF YOU HAVE NEVER EVEN CONSIDERED THE POSSIBILITY OF MENTAL IMMUNIZATION FROM ANY PARTICULAR DISEASE. AT ONE POINT IN YOUR HISTORY, THE MEN WHO CONSIDERED TRAVEL TO THE MOON WERE THOUGHT TO BE MAD, BUT NOW YOU ACCEPT THIS IDEA OF MOON TRAVEL AS FACT. WHEN I SPEAK ABOUT MENTAL IMMUNIZATION FROM ALL FORMS OF CANCER, OR DISEASE FOR THAT MATTER, I AM SPEAKING FROM AN EXPERIENCED STANDPOINT THAT YOU MIGHT

NOT SHARE. AFTER ALL, I AM A DOCTOR. YOUR PERSONAL PHYSICIAN AND I MIGHT HAVE A DIFFERENCE OF OPINION ON IMMUNIZATION AND EFFECTIVENESS OF MENTAL IMMUNIZATION. I ONCE SHARED THEIR VIEWS BUT HAVE SINCE CHANGED MY MIND ON THE SUBJECTS. YOU MAY ALSO CHANGE YOUR VIEWPOINT ON THE SUBJECT OF MENTAL IMMUNIZATION. CHANGE IS SOMETHING THAT WE ALL MUST LEARN TO ACCEPT. YOU DO NOT NOW HOLD THE SAME CHILDHOOD BELIEFS THAT YOU ONCE HELD. CHANGING YOUR MIND IS A SIGN OF DEVELOPMENT AND MATURITY. IT IS IMPORTANT THAT YOUR BELIEFS OR VIEWS BE TAKEN INTO CONSIDERATION AND CHANGED TO MORE BENEFICIAL VIEWS IF YOU ARE TO EFFECT IMMUNIZATION.

ACCEPTANCE OF THE IDEA OF BEING IMMUNE WILL CREATE THE IMMUNITY.

ACCEPTANCE OF A NEW IDEA IS ACHIEVED BY CONCENTRATING ON THE NEW IDEA FOR A TIME WITH THE MENTAL INTENTION THAT THIS IDEA BECOMES A PART OF YOUR BELIEF STRUCTURE. YOU BECOME IMMUNE FROM CANCER WHEN YOU ACCEPT THE IDEA THAT

*YOU ARE ALREADY IMMUNE FROM **ALL** FORMS OF CANCER AND HOLD NO VIEWS TO THE CONTRARY.*

IF A PERSON MAINTAINS THAT IMMUN-IZATION FROM ALL FORMS OF CANCER IS IMPOSSIBLE BY USING MENTAL TECHNIQUES, THEN IMMUNIZATION WILL BE IMPOSSIBLE BECAUSE OF THIS IDEA HE NOW HOLDS TO BE TRUE.

IT IS TRUE THAT YOUR THOUGHTS CREATE YOUR EXPERIENCES. FOLLOWING THIS LAW OF HUMAN BEHAVIOR, MY FIRST IMMUNIZATION TECHNIQUE THEN IS TO FOLLOW THOSE VIEWS WHICH YOU HOLD TO BE TRUE, WHICH KEEP YOU FROM CONTRACTING CANCER AND IGNORE OTHER VIEWS OR EVIDENCE. MY SECOND ALTERNATIVE IS TO ACCEPT THE IDEA THAT YOU ARE ALREADY IMMUNE FROM ALL FORMS OF CANCER AND HOLD NO VIEWS TO THE CON-TRARY. THE THIRD METHOD IS TO CHANGE THOSE VIEWS WHICH LEAD YOU TO BELIEVE YOU MIGHT CONTRACT CANCER AND INSTILL THE OPPOSITE IDEAS WHICH YOU ACCEPT AND WILL FOLLOW WHICH WILL PROTECT YOU FROM CANCER. THE LAST OF THE FOUR PERSONAL

IMMUNIZATION TECHNIQUES IS TO CHANGE THOSE VIEWS WHICH LEAD YOU TO BELIEVE YOU MIGHT GET CANCER AND ACCEPT THE IDEA YOU ARE ALREADY IMMUNE FROM ALL FORMS OF CANCER.

My next question to the doctor concerned the many individuals who have contracted cancer in spite of following recommended practices, which according to the doctor should have kept them from contracting cancer.

To this question came this reply: *FEARS ABOUT CONTRACTING CANCER IN ONE FORM OR ANOTHER, WHICH MANY OF THESE PEOPLE HELD, ARE ANOTHER FORM OF THE BELIEF THAT THEY WOULD CONTRACT CANCER AND THEY WERE HELPLESS TO HELP THEMSELVES IN THE FACE OF THIS DISEASE. WELL-INTENTIONED WARNINGS DID NOT HELP THE SITUATION AND, AS A MATTER OF FACT, DID CAUSE MORE PEOPLE TO CONTRACT THE DISEASE. UNLESS THESE FEARS ARE DEALT WITH SUCCESSFULLY IN WAYS I WILL PRESENT OR THROUGH OTHER MEANS, A CANCEROUS CONDITION MIGHT RESULT IN PEOPLE WHO HOLD TO THESE BELIEFS. FOLLOWING THE RULE THAT YOU MAY*

*READILY SEE THAT THESE FEARFUL SOULS AND
THOUGHTS CREATED THE CONDITIONS WHICH
PERMITTED THE EXPERIENCE OF CANCER.
THERE ARE OTHER EXPLANATIONS WHY A
PERSON MAY DECIDE TO CONTRACT CANCER
WHICH WILL HAVE TO BE DEALT WITH AT
ANOTHER TIME. IT IS NOT MY INTENTION TO
CAUSE AN INDIVIDUAL ANY UNDUE FEARS BY
IMPLYING THAT IF HE DOES NOT FOLLOW MY
PRESCRIPTION TO IMMUNIZE HIMSELF, HE WILL
CONTRACT CANCER. MY WORDS HERE ARE
INTENDED TO HELP THOSE WHO ALREADY HAVE
A FEAR OF CONTRACTING CANCER. THE
INDIVIDUALS WHO NOW TRULY CONSIDER
THEMSELVES IMMUNE FROM ANY TYPE OF
CANCER WILL NEVER CONTRACT CANCER. AS
LONG AS HE HOLDS THIS VIEW, HE WILL BE
IMMUNE FROM ALL FORMS OF CANCER.*

*THESE IMMUNITY PROCEDURES WILL WORK
AGAINST THE ACCEPTANCE OF ANY DISEASE. IF
THE CAUSE OF THE DISEASE IS EXTERNAL, THEN
THE CAUSES WILL BE AVOIDED. IF THE CAUSE
OF THE DISEASE IS INTERNAL OR INTERNALIZED,
THE MIND, WORKING THROUGH THE BODY,
WILL PROHIBIT THE MATERIALIZATION OF THE*

ILLNESS. IF AN EXTERNAL AGENT IS RESPONSIBLE, WHICH IS NOT POSSIBLE TO AVOID, THEN THE BODY WILL HAVE BUILT UP A DEFENSE SYSTEM, SECOND TO NONE, WHICH WILL NOT BE BROKEN DOWN. GOOD HEALTH WILL CONTINUE FOR AS LONG AS THE INDIVIDUAL CONTINUES TO MAINTAIN THAT HE IS IMMUNE FROM A PARTICULAR DISEASE.

INDIVIDUALS HAVE REACHED A STAGE OF DEVELOPMENT WHERE ACCEPTANCE OF IMMUNITY FROM ALL DISEASE IS POSSIBLE. THE FIRST EXPERIENCES OF IMMUNITY FROM ALL DISEASE WILL BE, OF COURSE, ON AN INDIVIDUAL BASIS, BEFORE SOCIETY OR GROUPS WITHIN SOCIETY EXPERIENCE IMMUNITY FROM ALL DISEASES. THE SEEDS OF THIS IDEA WILL BE HARVESTED LATER IN YOUR TIME ZONE BY LARGE SEGMENTS OF THE POPULACE. I SAY THIS TO YOU BECAUSE THE POTENTIAL EXISTS FOR SUCH ACTIVITY NOW. NO ONE HOLDS BACK ANY GROUP FROM SUCH LINES OF DEVELOPMENT. IT IS INDIVIDUALS AND GROUPS WHO NOW HOLD MAN BACK FROM THIS EXPERIENCE BECAUSE OF THEIR BELIEFS. FACTORS WILL CAUSE THESE BELIEFS TO

CHANGE. ONE IDEA WHICH KEEPS THIS LINE OF IMMUNIZATION FROM BEING EXPERIENCED NOW IS THE VIEW THAT PHYSICAL REALITY IS LESS DESIROUS THAN OTHER NON-PHYSICAL REALITIES. THIS IS NOT THE CASE. THIS IDEA FOSTERS THE VIEW THAT MAN IS SOMEHOW BEING PUNISHED FOR HIS OWN IMAGINED TRANSGRESSIONS OR THE IMAGINED TRANSGRESSIONS OF OTHERS. THIS IS NOT TRUE. ANOTHER VIEW WHICH HOLDS MAN BACK FROM THIS LINE OF DEVELOPMENT IS HIS FALSE IDEA OF JUSTICE. TRUE JUSTICE IS NOT FOSTERED WHEN ANY FORM OF PUNISHMENT IS ADMINISTERED BY OUTSIDE FORCES.

IT IS AN INDIVIDUAL'S DUTY TO HIMSELF TO USE ANY MEANS SHORT OF VIOLENCE TO ESCAPE OR AVOID PUNISHMENT.

WHOEVER IS CLAIMING THE AUTHORITY TO PUNISH ANOTHER OR TO HARM ANOTHER IS MAKING A FALSE CLAIM. NO BEING OR LAW GIVES ANYONE THE RIGHT TO PUNISH OR HARM ANOTHER. SELF-DEFENSE DOES NOT JUSTIFY KILLING OR HARMING ANOTHER PERSON. THERE EXISTS NO JUSTIFICATION FOR ANY PUNISHMENT IN PHYSICAL OR NON-PHYSICAL

REALITIES. HEAVEN-OR-HADES CONDITIONS IN NON-PHYSICAL REALITIES ARE TEMPORARY CONDITIONS, IF EXPERIENCED, WHICH NO OUTSIDE BEINGS OR BEING FORCES UPON ANOTHER.

MY EXISTENCE AND EXPERIENCES IN PHYSICAL REALITIES SIMILAR TO YOURS SHOW CONCLUSIVELY THAT A NO PUNISHMENT ENVIRONMENT IS A BETTER ALTERNATIVE THAN THE ONE YOU ARE NOW WORKING WITH.

OTHER BELIEFS WHICH ARE HOLDING BACK MAN FROM FOLLOWING A DIFFERENT LINE OF DEVELOPMENT WHICH WOULD INCLUDE IMMUNITY FROM ALL DISEASES ARE HIS REAL GUILT FROM ARTIFICIAL LAWS AND THE IDEA THAT THE BODY IS WEAK IN THE FACE OF DISEASE OR IS SUBJECT TO ILLNESS OVER WHICH HE HAS NO CONTROL. IDEAS SUCH AS THESE KEEP MAN FROM EXPERIENCING IMMUNITY AS A GROUP. NO ONE FORCES ANYTHING ON YOU. YOU HAVE ACCEPTED THESE IDEAS WITHOUT QUESTION. THOSE PERSONS IN YOUR TIME ZONE WHO WILL EXIST IN THE FUTURE AND YOU, THE READER, MAY BE ONE AMONG THAT NUMBER WHO WILL HAVE

DIFFERENT EXPERIENCES THAN ARE NOW POSSIBLE. THOSE OF YOU WHO AWAIT THE "SECOND COMING OF CHRIST" WILL FIND THIS "CHRIST-FIGURE PERSONALITY" DESTROY WHAT REMAINS OF HIS CHURCH.

EDUCATION PROCESSES WILL THEN INCLUDE TECHNIQUES TO ACHIEVE IMMUNITY AS A NATURAL OUTGROWTH OF HUMAN POTENTIAL. SOME MEN NOW ATTEMPT THROUGH RE-EDUCATION TO START THIS PROGRAM. INDIVIDUAL TRAINING WITHIN THE FAMILY STRUCTURE ABOUT THE TRUE CAUSES OF DISEASE AND IMMUNITY WILL BE AN IMPORTANT FACTOR IN THIS DEVELOPMENTAL AND EDUCATIONAL PROCESS.

As you can see from what the doctor said on immunization, if you do not already consider yourself immune from all forms of cancer, there must be a change of your views to one that is more beneficial. For example, if you now hold to the idea that mental immunization is impossible, you will have to effect a change of view. One method I have used successfully to change my view has been to apply the same means which you may already use to change something about your life you do not like. I called this method the effective wishful thinking technique.

In this method you must first objectify (by writing down) all your ideas which lead you to believe mental immunization is impossible. From those opinions, identify the main or pivotal ideas. Now, once you identify the main idea as something you no longer accept, your other subordinate ideas will follow suit. For example, from among all your opinions, you may feel the main idea is that mental immunization is impossible. Alongside the main idea, put down the new outlook you would like to have, which is that mental immunization is possible. By applying the effective wishful thinking technique to what you have written, you should be able to come up with your own formula for changing this main idea and other ideas you hold to a more hopeful view.

My sentences looked like this, although yours may vary: "The views I held about mental immunization being impossible were a part of my personality. Now in this new instance I realize mental immunization is possible." For a period each day, dwell on your new opinion, which will soon become a part of your belief structure. Within a month, the sentences which you used to state a new, clear, mental intention should take hold and then you are ready to take the next step in immunizing yourself against all forms of cancer.

The object of the next step is to effect any one of the four alternatives that the doctor recommended. I would say that a person should select the one alternative that he feels best suits his personality and needs. If the ones provided do not suit your needs, you may wish to design your own mental immunization program against cancer.

The first alternative suggested by the doctor is, "Follow those views which you hold to be true which keep you from contracting cancer and ignore other views or evidence." When I state my mental intention, using the effective wishful thinking technique, I come up with these sentences.

Your sentence structure may differ. It is your mental intention that is important and not the exact wording of the sentences. "I direct that I follow those views that I already hold to be true which will keep me from contracting all forms of cancer. I further direct that I ignore all other views or evidence." By accepting this mental intention as a part of your belief structure, for a period not to exceed a month in most instances, a person will have effectively protected himself against all forms of cancer.

Acceptance of the new view is achieved by

dwelling on this mental intention daily for a short time. By way of further explanation the doctor feels it important that I now add this: *IT IS NOT MY INTENTION THAT YOU SHOULD BURY YOUR HEAD IN THE SAND FROM CONTRARY VIEWS TO MINE ABOUT CANCER. BUT AS A PRACTICAL MATTER, IT IS BETTER FOR MOST INDIVIDUALS WHO UNDERTAKE A MENTAL IMMUNIZATION PROGRAM TO IGNORE OTHER VIEWS, EVIDENCE, OR FINDINGS TO THE CONTRARY, FOR A PERIOD OF TIME AND AT LEAST FOR THAT PERIOD OF TIME WHICH MIGHT BE REQUIRED TO FIND EVIDENCE TO FURTHER SUPPORT YOURSELF IN YOUR NEW CONVICTION THAT YOU ARE INDEED IMMUNE FROM ALL TYPES OF CANCER.*

As you will recall from a remark made earlier by the doctor about the causes of cancer, he said, "There must be an acceptance of the disease by the individual. The individual permits the physical experience of this disease and every disease for their own personal reasons." The doctor is now recommending a practical way where acceptance of the disease is not permitted. This intention is the first line of defense against cancer.

The second alternative suggested by the doctor is

"accept the idea you are already immune from all forms of cancer and hold no views to the contrary." In addition to the first line of defense, a second line of defense is created by the body. The second line of defense is the creation by the body of natural antibodies against all forms of the disease, while the first line of defense, which is non-acceptance of the disease by the individual, is maintained. This is the alternative that I selected to use for myself.

First, I objectified my views and declared my mental intention using the same wishful thinking technique I illustrated previously. I arrived at this sentence: "I direct that I am already immune from all forms of cancer and hold no views to the contrary." Then by dwelling on or repeating this same sentence to myself early in the morning, which I have found to be the best time for me to rid myself of the beliefs I do not want and to accept new views, I started to become immune.

My idea of dwelling on a new mental intention is to repeat the sentence to myself several times. Then say the same sentence louder to myself a few more times. Then I would say each word slowly and very deliberately while thinking about the meaning of each word in this clear mental intention I constructed.

Sometimes I vary the wording so I don't get bored with the mental exercise. I recognize that it is my mental intention that deals with eliminating negative ideas and creating new positive ideas that is important and not the exact wording. When I get comfortable with a particular phraseology, I keep at it until I feel sure I accepted this new belief as a part of my personal belief structure. I did not tell any of my friends what I was doing until after I had completed the program. By then, immunization was an accomplished fact and a part of my belief structure. After adjustments, to suit my personality and to find a phraseology that I was comfortable with, I ended up with this direction: "I direct that I suspend all views I hold in the area of cancer. I direct that I am already immune from all forms of cancer and hold no views to the contrary."

Because I had accepted the idea that most diseases are caused by some psychological factors, I had no built-in resistance to overcome before starting my own personal immunization program. Acceptance of this new idea was easy. On the other hand, I was disappointed that I did not first think of the idea myself. It seems rather odd for me to say that, since the idea sprang through me.

As funny as it may sound, I sometimes post new

ideas I want to have in the bathroom. The time I spend in the bathroom in the morning coincides with the amount of time I require to accept a new idea. I post the paper in a conspicuous place so I will not forget to do the exercise daily. This is the one place in my home where I am least likely to be distracted or disturbed.

It was not a coincidence, according to the doctor, that I had a slight case of diarrhea when I first started doing the mental exercise. Before anyone else feels that in order for the immunization program to be effective, he must have a slight case of diarrhea, let me assure you this is not the case. A slight case of diarrhea was my personal way of assuring myself that there was a physical reaction to my mental immunization program. You may or may not have the same reaction.

The third alternative the doctor presented was, "Change those views that lead you to believe that you might contract cancer, and instill opposite ideas that you accept and will follow, which will protect you from cancer." For example, if you believe you will contract cancer from cigars, cigarettes, or pipe-smoking, you must change this idea you hold to one that you will not contract any form of cancer from smoking cigars, cigarettes, or pipe-smoking. When I reduce this example to our effective wishful thinking technique, I arrive at these sentences which clearly formulate my mental intention. "I direct that the views I hold about contracting cancer through smoking were a part of my personality. Now, in this new instance, I accept the idea that smoking is not harmful to my health." The idea of immunity is implied in this exercise by changing your viewpoints about what might cause you to contract cancer.

Should you at any time find your mind drifting from these exercises and want to follow another thought, follow that thought to its conclusion and then come back to the exercise.

The fourth alternative that the doctor presented was, "Change those views that lead you to believe you might get cancer, and accept the idea that you are immune from all forms of cancer." By way of illustration, if you believe cancer is hereditary and a member of your family has had cancer, it will be necessary for you to change this view that leads you to believe you might get cancer and accept the new idea you want.

Our first step, again, is to objectify our viewpoints. Write down on a piece of paper those negative ideas you have. Some will want to put the paper aside for a while to see if any other negative ideas come to mind. Next, alongside those negative remarks, write down opposite, or positive ideas.

Then, immediately following your negative views about contracting cancer, you might add this statement: "These views and opinions were a part of my personality. They are a part of my old belief structure that I no longer accept. Instead, I choose to follow and accept these more beneficial beliefs." (Here insert your more positive and beneficial views.) Then add, "I also choose to accept that fact I am now immune from all forms of cancer. I hold no views to the contrary."

When we draw up our new mental direction, it may look something similar to this: "I suggest these views I have that cancer is hereditary or may be contracted from smoking are opinion. These opinions and views were a part of my personality. They are a part of my old belief structure that I no longer accept; instead, I choose to follow and accept these more beneficial beliefs. Cancer is not hereditary. Smoking does not cause cancer. I also choose to accept the fact I am now already immune from all forms of cancer. I hold no views to the contrary."

The theme behind all the alternatives presented is to replace all negative views that you might have about contracting cancer with more beneficial views. In any program that you devise, be sure to first deal with the negative ideas and then instill positive beliefs. Should you enlist the help of a friend to formulate your personal program, remember you are the final judge of what is best for you. Follow your own feelings and quiet thoughts on what best suits your personality. Your friend may be unwittingly projecting his requirements for his personal program on what he feels you need to do to effect an immunization program.

All four personal mental immunization programs in most instances should not take more than a month to be effective. If you feel safer prolonging the exercise, do so. The doctor would now like to add the following: *IT MAY BE NECESSARY FOR THOSE WHO HAVE UNDERTAKEN THE PROGRAM OF MENTAL IMMUNIZATION TO PERIODICALLY REVIEW THE ALTERNATIVE THEY HAVE SELECTED TO USE. THIS WILL INSURE THAT, FOR ONE REASON OR ANOTHER, THE FACT THEY ARE IMMUNE FROM ALL FORMS OF CANCER HAS NOT LOST ITS FOOTING. YOUR IMMUNITY WILL LAST AS LONG AS YOU BELIEVE YOU ARE IMMUNE AND HOLD NO VIEWS TO THE CONTRARY.*

ANY VIEWS TO THE CONTRARY YOU ACCEPT AT A LATER DATE MUST BE DEALT WITH AGAIN BY USING ANY OF THE ALTERNATIVE IMMUNIZATION PROGRAMS PRESENTED. THIS WILL INSURE YOUR IMMUNITY PROCEDURES HAVE NOT BEEN SHORT-CIRCUITED. THIS HOLDS TRUE FOR ANY DISEASE AGAINST WHICH YOU WISH TO IMMUNIZE YOURSELF BY USING THESE PROCEDURES.

THERE WILL COME A TIME WHEN THE PROCEDURES RECOMMENDED WILL BE TESTED BY MEDICAL AUTHORITIES. SHOULD THEIR FINDINGS CONFLICT WITH MY OPINIONS, YOU WILL HAVE TO DETERMINE FOR YOURSELF WHAT YOU WILL ACCEPT AS BEING TRUE. AT THAT TIME, INSTANCES IN WHICH IMMUNITY BY INDIVIDUALS WAS NOT ACHIEVED AGAINST ALL FORMS OF CANCER WILL REFLECT THAT THOSE PERSONS DID NOT TRULY CONSIDER THEMSELVES IMMUNE FROM ALL FORMS OF CANCER. THE CAUSE WILL BE A FAILURE TO CONSIDER ALL THEIR NEGATIVE UNEXAMINED BELIEFS WHICH LED TO HIDDEN FEARS ABOUT CONTRACTING CANCER. THE WORDS "HIDDEN FEARS" INDICATE BELIEFS LEADING TO THOSE

FEARS WHICH WERE UNEXAMINED, BUT NOT HIDDEN FROM VIEW.

I DO NOT MEAN HERE TO BE NEGATIVE ABOUT THE PROGRAMS I HAVE JUST RECOMMENDED YOU FOLLOW. I MUST BE A REALIST. NOT EVERYONE WILL SUCCESSFULLY UNDERTAKE THESE PROGRAMS, NOR WILL EVERYONE TAKE THE NECESSARY STEPS TO CORRECT THE CONTRARY VIEWS THEY LATER ACCEPT ABOUT CONTRACTING CANCER AFTER EFFECTIVELY IMMUNIZING THEMSELVES FOR A TIME AGAINST CANCER. AS ANY OTHER DOCTOR WILL TELL YOU, PATIENTS DO NOT ALWAYS FOLLOW PRESCRIPTIONS TO AVOID CONTRACTING DISEASES. NO MATTER HOW SIMPLE THE STEPS OR HOW LITTLE TIME THE IMMUNIZATION STEPS TAKE.

The last immunization procedures I learned about are designed to produce immunity against cancer or other diseases in other individuals who are unable to undertake a personal immunization program themselves. In this procedure, the power of one individual to influence another individual is recognized. One of the mental immunization procedures learned was *VISUALIZE YOUR FRIEND AS BEING IMMUNE*

FROM ALL FORMS OF CANCER.

In this alternative, you mentally support an individual to conform to your new view of him. The individual involved ultimately decides whether or not to conform to your new view of him. No individual or being has the power to harm another person by the power of his thoughts. Likewise, no person, by the power of his thoughts, can cause a person to act, even in a beneficial way. You cannot force a person to change his views, but your expectations can influence him telepathically to accept certain ideas as opposed to less beneficial beliefs. You follow the wishful thinking techniques that you feel fit the situation, only now he becomes the subject.

First, take into consideration any negative ideas you hold about why this person might contract cancer by listing them on a piece of paper. You then decide to deal with these negative views in a manner chosen from any of the alternatives presented earlier. Or you may decide to use the following sentence to objectify your mental intention: "All those negative views I held about my friend contracting cancer were a part of my attitude. Now in this new instance I see my friend as being immune from all forms of cancer." This last sentence presented objectifies your mental intention to visualize your friend as being immune from all forms of cancer.

The closer your personal or psychic relationship, the more likely your friend will be influenced by your thoughts. The doctor states, *SOME MENTAL SUPPORT IS BETTER THAN NO SUPPORT AT ALL OR VIEWS TO THE CONTRARY THAT YOUR FRIEND MIGHT GET CANCER.*

When you feel you have changed the way you pictured your friend to a more hopeful picture, stop this exercise. He will telepathically get the message and it will be his responsibility to act or not act on your new picture of him.

The doctor would like to add a comment regarding persons who may read this and not act for the benefit of a friend, for one reason or another: *NO INDIVIDUAL SHOULD FEEL GUILTY OR HAVE PANGS OF CONSCIENCE FOR FAILING TO ACT TELEPATHICALLY TO IMMUNIZE A FRIEND. YOUR FRIEND HAS DECIDED TO CONTRACT CANCER FOR HIS OWN PERSONAL REASONS. HIS CONDITION SHOULD NOT BE ACCEPTED AS A REASON FOR YOU TO FEEL GUILTY.*

This last alternative also includes directions to be used with persons who rely on other people for guidance and with children. The doctor now wishes to say: *PERSONS WHO ARE DEPENDENT UPON OTHERS FOR GUIDANCE AND CHILDREN SHOULD BE TOLD THEY ARE IMMUNE FROM ALL FORMS OF CANCER. CHILDREN WHO ARE TOLD THEY ARE IMMUNE FROM ALL FORMS OF CANCER WILL IMMUNIZE THEMSELVES SUCCESSFULLY AGAINST ALL FORMS OF CANCER BECAUSE, FOR A TIME, CHILDREN ACCEPT VIEWS HELD BY PARENTS AND OTHER AUTHORITY FIGURES. THIS ALSO HOLDS TRUE FOR PERSONS WHO RELY UPON OTHERS FOR GUIDANCE. IMMUNITY WILL LAST AS LONG AS THE BELIEF STRUCTURES REMAIN INTACT. YOUNG ADULTS WHO HAVE BEEN IMMUNIZED FROM A PARTICULAR DISEASE OR FROM ALL FORMS OF CANCER BY ACCEPTING THE BELIEFS OF PARENTS, FRIENDS, OR OTHER AUTHORITY FIGURES, MAY WISH TO REINFORCE THIS BELIEF STRUCTURE FOR THEMSELVES AT A LATER DATE.*

THE OBJECT OF THE EXERCISES THAT WERE SHOWN IS THE CONSTRUCTION OF THE BELIEF THAT A PERSON IS IMMUNE FROM ALL FORMS OF CANCER. FROM THIS CORE OR MAIN IDEA

131

WILL SPRING OTHER IDEAS THAT WILL SUPPORT HIM IN THIS NEW CONVICTION. HE WILL NOW FIND NEW EVIDENCE TO SUPPORT HIMSELF IN THIS CONVICTION. JUST AS EASILY AS HE FOUND REASONS TO BELIEVE THAT HE MIGHT CONTRACT CANCER, NOW HE WILL FIND REASONS TO SUPPORT THE OPPOSITE VIEW.

THE IMMUNIZATION PROCEDURES DISCUSSED WILL WORK WITH DISEASES YET UNNAMED.

Chapter Five

LEARNING ABOUT
THE "UNKNOWN"

When I began to consider writing this story of a cancer cure, I decided the most important element of the story was not the cure itself or even the immunization procedures. I decided the most important element of the story should be the documentation of the mental processes that led to the discoveries. Here, I reasoned, was a key which could open up the door to other discoveries by individuals in their own field of interest.

With self-training, any person could duplicate the procedures used to learn about the nature of cancer. My experience in learning something new was not unique. The same process I used I am sure has been used in the past. However, what was unusual was that I understood the process on a conscious level.

I reasoned, at the time my first psychic inquiries

about cancer began, that the answer was probably known somewhere in the system. I realized ideas do not exist in a vacuum. So there must be a container, even if this container is invisible to our physical eyes. The container of this information I sought was a doctor, although, at the time, I did not know this fact. I am of the opinion that anyone who is interested enough in learning about new ideas can do so, using the method I propose, without needing to know the identity of the provider of the information or even that this information is learned by telepathic means. Before I present this material on the origin of ideas, I think it would be better for those interested individuals to first become familiar with the origins of their own ideas and personal answer bank. However, a working knowledge of your inner logic system is not required to learn data from an external answer bank.

I am going to use analogies to present the general background information on directly using your personal answer bank. I will avoid using the terms that you may use to describe the functions and parts of the mind because our meanings may differ. I will detail specific steps that a person may use to become acquainted with the content of his data bank, if he is not already aware of the methods involved.

The same methods may be used by persons who are interested in developing either mental or physical talents, in addition to the ones they have already developed. I will be providing some basic tools and concepts to develop new talents that a person will be expected to adapt to suit his personality and needs. The one new talent I will use to illustrate how all new talents may be developed is the ability to learn answers directly from your personal answer bank.

Already you are learning answers to your personal questions from your data bank. You may not now even be aware of this fact. The answers to our questions are sometimes presented in such an indirect fashion that we do not know we are providing ourselves with these answers. As a result of your developing an ability to learn answers directly from this bank of ideas, you may begin to consciously explore its contents. There are many ways an individual may learn of the contents. I am going to present a method that I propose you test to see if it suits your needs.

The method you may now be using to become aware of your own information center I am going to call the intellectual or indirect approach. The method I propose you try is the intuitive, or direct approach. The difference is not in the end product, but rather in the way the end product or information may be arrived at. For example, the reasons why you have decided to occupy this body at this point in time is known to you right now.

If you desire this information, there are clues you are now presenting to yourself. Using your intellectual powers, you could put together the clues and arrive at those reasons. By using your intuitive abilities, which you can develop, and taking advantage of your inner logic system, you may learn the reasons directly. How you arrive at those reasons or what might now be "unknown" to a part of you is what this chapter is about.

The cornerstone of establishing a direct channel from your answer bank, if this is the mental talent you wish to develop, will be based upon the acceptance of this one pivotal idea: Expecting an answer, ask yourself the question. A person will learn information directly from his data bank after he first expects his questions to be answered. Likewise, a person interested in learning new ideas from an external answer bank will learn the data when he first expects his questions to be answered. Other mental or physical talents, from telepathy to playing baseball, will be based upon the acceptance of different pivotal ideas. You create the ability to answer questions by first convincing yourself you can learn the answers before you ever ask the questions.

This observation, that a person must first expect to have his questions answered before asking the question, was made after friends tried to obtain answers to their questions from their information center using the same questioning techniques I used but did not get good results. Had these same friends first convinced themselves of their ability to answer questions, the results would have been different.

My chief concern at this point is the laying of a good foundation that will enable persons to develop the talents they want. In order to lay a good foundation, I will have to deal with some of the ideas that you now hold to be true. I will discuss attitudes and their formation. I will also touch upon some of the operations of your mind. The process of developing talents will include: a point by point discussion of your sleep patterns, specific dream directions, removing blockages to talent development, substituting one pivotal idea for another, and a practical illustration by which these techniques may be used to change a situation with which you are not happy.

The specific methods I present are not expected to

exactly fit everyone's needs because we all are different. The differences in who we are and what we think may make a method suitable for me but unsuitable for your needs. If you do elect to try the alternatives, it is recommended that you test them for only an initial two- or three-month period. If you are not successful, do not pull your hair out trying to make something work which is not suited to your personality. You may do yourself more harm than good. At some later point in time, you may wish to try again.

If you are successful in learning answers directly from your answer bank after the initial testing period, it is strongly recommended that you become familiar with its contents for at least a two-year period before trying the more advanced psychic techniques dealing with the origin of ideas.

You do not have to learn or master the alternatives I am suggesting here to develop new talents or to obtain information from your data bank to immunize yourself from all forms of cancer. All interested persons are expected to be able to achieve immunity using those steps I have already provided. Testing of this alternative I propose should follow the month or so it will take to immunize yourself from all forms of cancer.

In presenting this material, stress will be placed upon proper attitude formation. Some recommended exercises are meant to be followed and used. I have found these basic exercises work best to create proper attitudes.

A change of attitudes and views is necessary for those who are not already experiencing direct levels of communication with their information center. Attitudes are a collection of ideas we hold about a subject. An attitude usually centers around one main pivotal idea. For example, a new pivotal idea that you may hold is the view that you can be immune from all forms of cancer. This main or pivotal idea may be later supported by subordinate ideas. You may observe that not all persons contract cancer; therefore, some psychological factors must be at work.

I will be asking you to pay close attention to the pivotal ideas that you hold about certain subjects so that you may identify the main reasons for your different attitudes. A subordinate idea for one person may be the main or pivotal idea for another. Where appropriate, I will suggest certain new pivotal ideas to effect a change in your attitudes.

Because of the many different attitudes all of us

have that are based upon strong convictions, no single formula or alternative I propose is going to establish a direct channel from everyone's information center. There is no single magic door, just as there is no single magic door for a successful-formula for raising kids, for marriage, or for business. It will be more to your credit if you are able to adapt my alternative to fit your personality, than to my credit for providing the alternative.

A game-like "I'll-try-it" attitude and a sense of humor will work better for you over the long haul. Enjoying what you are doing will keep you interested. If you don't like the new adventure, or if it grows distasteful, then in all probability you will quit. It will also be to your advantage to know there are no rules to this game of developing an ability to learn answers to your personal questions directly. Only guidelines are presented. You win the game when you prove to yourself my contention that you can directly utilize your answer bank. Some readers will already recognize, from their past experience, the existence of this inner source of knowledge and may now wish to establish a more direct channel.

You will have to have a certain amount of maturity to deal with quiet thoughts. Those who do experience quiet thoughts, however unusual, will be prepared to handle them or they would not permit the experience in the first place. For example, let us say you have already developed the ability to obtain answers, and you ask why you have a sore throat. You learn you have a sore throat because you are afraid to tell the truth to an associate about his offensive breath odor. In addition to a certain maturity needed to deal with this learning, you will also have to have flexibility. Flexibility will be needed to act upon the information and correct the situation. The answers you provide yourself with are intended to be acted upon, as you would expect your associate to do something about his offensive breath odor.

If you are not satisfied with a proposed course of action that you learn about through quiet thoughts, you should now recognize your answer bank is designed to provide you with more than one practical choice to suit your needs. Different alternatives may be requested. Not just one course of action must be followed. You always have the choice to follow or not to follow a quiet thought. Let us say you have asked yourself how you can resolve a marriage problem. You learn that you could take a two week "get-away-from-it-all" vacation from your husband and kids. You decide not

142

to follow this thought. So you ask for a different choice. Now you learn that you could for the next six months spend two nights a week visiting friends. Still not satisfied, you ask again. You learn a nightly hour walk by yourself will give you the solitude you require away from your family to "recharge your batteries." This thought you decide to follow.

The methods I propose may serve to confirm a viewpoint you already hold (although you may not express it in the same way I do), or the methods may challenge your viewpoints. Deciding not to accept my viewpoints may be better for you than holding on to your own opposing viewpoints and at the same time accepting my views. You will cause yourself some degree of anxiety. It is recommended strongly that you test these opposing views and then, on the basis of your own conclusions, decide which to accept and follow.

You are being invited in this chapter to test the capability of your own information center. Its capacity for learning is unlimited, and hence the capacity for dissemination of information learned is likewise unlimited. It will be easier for a person to prove to himself that he can solve family, work, love, business, and health problems by using his information center than to prove the validity of certain other capacities. For example, the subjective knowledge available in any one individual's personal answer bank is enough to re-create entire worlds. Likewise, the subjective knowledge contained in a drop of water is sufficient to create this entire universe anew.

Despite this tremendous reserve of knowledge available to an individual, it is not expected that a person will learn how to solve all his problems overnight. It is expected that you will opt to work for a gradual development as you begin to deal with your quiet thoughts. The methods will call for more introspection on the reader's part, but not for all introspection.

The methods are designed to alert you to your own innate capability for intuitive rather than intellectual learning. I would like to present an analogy to make my point clearer. When I think about resolving problems or challenges, I think of them as moves in chess. When I play chess, I am using a part of my intellectual capabilities to make the right moves. If my opponent makes a certain move, then I will move my piece to a certain position. If he moves a different piece, I use my reasoning capabilities to come up with another move. When I think about what I should do to solve problems in life, I also use my reasoning or intellectual capabilities.

Now, like the moves in life, the game of chess has long been thought to be better played by persons using only intellectual powers. However, when I play the game of chess, or life, I also use innate quiet thoughts or intuitive abilities. I combine the two different operations involved in reasoning and intuition to make moves. You cannot tell from the outside which operation I am using, but I do use both and have tried to create a balance.

When I am stuck for a move in chess, or life, I literally ask myself for the next move from my personal answer bank. In chess, and in life, after a time, I developed the ability to have the intuitive move there in seconds. I became aware of an answer in the form of a quiet thought. I am using a portion of the same innate intuitive logic system which gives rise to the physical system that controls the flow of blood to play chess and make decisions in life. Compared to the thousands of calculations a part of you makes every moment just to maintain your body, a chess move is simple. I hope my true analogy gives the reader a hint of his tremendous inner problem-solving capabilities which he already has available to him. A person who maintains a balance between this intuitive and intellectual problem-solving capabilities develops an ingoing and outgoing personality.

Had a doctor made a discovery about the use of heather to cure certain types of cancer, he probably would have credited his intellectual problem-solving capabilities. If this imaginary doctor had decided to test a thousand different natural products directly on patients and had eliminated all products except heather as being useless, the doctor's learning would have been the result of an intellectual process. He would have had to sift through the data from his externally perceived experiments, analyze the information, and come to conclusions. He would have arrived at this conclusion about heather from physically perceived external sense data.

On the other hand, I arrived at my conclusions using an intuitive process. I sifted through the data from inner non-physically perceived quiet thought experiments, analyzed the information, and came to a conclusion. I arrived at my conclusions about heather by using non-physical perception capabilities of inner sense data. The conclusions reached by our imaginary doctor and myself would have been the same. Both the intellectual and intuitive methods are valid means of making discoveries or making conclusions. But the methods, as you can see from this illustration, are different.

The different methods used by our imaginary doctor and myself result from using different faculties of the brain. The brain, in turn, is only capable of using these different faculties because of the different capabilities and operations of the mind. This does not mean that one method is superior to the other. The roots of a tree are not superior to the branches of the tree. Intuitive or quiet thought learning is not superior to intellectual processes. Nor is reasoning or intellectual learning superior to intuitive processes. However, it is valid to say that by and large man has not developed intuitive processes to the extent that intellectual processes have been developed.

When I think about the mind, I am reminded of an analogy I use to help me understand how the mind functions. I think of an imaginary egg. The shell of the egg represents my physical container or body. The white of the egg represents my intellectual processes. These are the processes that deal directly with physical reality. This part of the mind sifts through data from seeing and hearing and arrives at certain conclusions. I call this part of my mind "the lesser reality."

Another part of my mind is represented by the yolk or yellow of the egg. This part represents my intuitive processes. These processes deal with non-physical reality. This part of the mind, among other duties, sifts through data when we dream and arrives at certain conclusions. I call this creation or part of my mind my "greater reality."

By using the terms lesser and greater realities, I am not saying one is superior to the other. I use the different terms to remind me that the lesser reality is a creation of the greater reality. Following the example of our imaginary egg, we can see that the yellow of the egg appears to create the white of the egg, and together both appear to create and maintain the shell. Said another way, the greater reality gives rise to the lesser reality, and together both create and maintain our bodies.

Using our egg analogy again, we can better realize how ultimately our individual physical structures evolve from a non-physical structure called the mind.

The separate functions of the lesser reality (dealing with physical sensory data) and the greater reality (dealing with one's non-physical inner sense data) do exist. However, the divisions of the mind as such, represented by the different parts of the egg, do not exist. A closer picture of what the mind is would be better represented, using our egg analogy, by a scrambled egg still within the shell.

The different functions of the lesser reality and the greater reality result in different characteristics and, fortunate for us, peculiarities. For example, the lesser reality pretends not to know what the greater reality knows. So what is already known by a part of us is "unknown" by another part. In a very real sense, the greater reality plays the children's game of "come and find me." And the lesser reality pretends not to know where to look.

The game is played by individuals for variations on the same general theme. We present challenges to ourselves with the knowing consent of our greater reality to be experienced by the lesser reality. Thus, necessary developmental lessons will be learned in physical reality that would not otherwise be possible. One important lesson is that our thoughts create our experiences. This lesson can be expressed in another way: "to see your thoughts materialized in physical reality." I am, of course, giving a very broad, general overview. The particular reasons for your being in physical reality are already known by your greater reality, even though your lesser reality may pretend not to know, is illustrative of the point I am trying to make here.

Now, for the white of the egg or lesser reality to learn directly what the yellow of the egg or greater reality already knows takes time. The developmental process of the white of the egg is gradual because it must deal with physical reality and follow certain rules. For this reason it is not expected that a person will open a direct channel to or from his answer bank overnight.

Your lesser reality, which operates so efficiently during the times you are awake to deal in physical reality, moves aside during sleep periods for your greater reality to take over the controls. Those of you who have developed the ability to become awake in your dreams are aware of this. It is your greater reality that was pushed aside during the day that now controls what happens in your dreams. Now the lesser reality is not shut off entirely when you sleep, but you do focus your attention elsewhere. Likewise, when you are awake your greater reality still functions, but you are not generally aware of its functions at the time because you are so busy dealing with physical reality.

The greater reality controls what happens when you dream. A dream is one form of a non-physical event. To your greater reality, non-physical events are as real as physical events are to your lesser reality. It may be that you are only aware of the fact that your mind continues to function because of a nightmare which you recall having. I am reminding you that your mind works at night because one step of the process I will propose you try does involve using the sleep state. We are going to suggest you put your greater reality to work in a certain direction while your body rests. You will not be asked to remember the dream or give an interpretation. You will be asked to only give certain directions by using one or two-sentence instructions.

To illustrate how your greater reality functions at night for those readers who are not aware of what happens when you think you are "asleep," let us say you want to solve a particular work-related problem. You want to know how to deal with an employee or manager at work. So you ask yourself a question, expecting an answer, just before you go to sleep. Your lesser reality which gave the instruction now moves aside and lets the greater reality solve the problem. The latter may trigger a certain memory from a similar past experience in which you successfully dealt with a similar problem. Or it may decide to work out new alternative solutions to choose which one works best.

For example, because your non-physical body is not limited by the time and space limits of your physical body, you may act with the non-physical bodies of others in working out the different solutions.

It may be possible for you to physically perceive with your own naked eyesight the non-physical or astral body of another person. Our more stouthearted psychic explorers may wish to develop an ability to become aware of non-physical bodies by applying principles discussed in this chapter. I once told a friend, who lives in a different town, that each night we all take side-trips using our astral bodies for a period of time, although we are not all consciously alert to our nightly travels. She decided, without telling me beforehand, to give herself a suggestion just before she went to sleep to visit me in her astral body. When I became aware of her presence in my room, I awoke from my sleep. I remember saying to her out loud, "Oh, it's only you." Then I went back to sleep. In the morning I gave her a call to confirm for her that her specific astral body dream suggestion to visit me did result in a visit. She did not consciously remember the dream or the visit but did recall making the dream suggestion to pay me a visit.

Once your greater reality has decided on which

alternative to use during sleep, it must now present the information to the lesser reality or ego. At the end of the interpretive process, the ego knows what it is going to do to solve the problem at work.

Now, you may or may not know at the ego level that the solution was decided upon by your greater reality while you slept. You may not even recall having the dream. It may be in the morning or sometime during the day that you will have a quiet thought that you will act upon. You may even credit your intellectual process with giving you the answer, but the true credit belongs to your greater reality. Every night when you sleep you act out what you are going to do when you are awake. Persons who have a feeling of being in a place or doing an activity before are recalling these dream events. It may also be that your greater reality will have to use more circuitous routes to shape events to remind you of the solution you decided upon the night before. Now your greater reality not only functions behind the scenes when you are awake to form physical events but also stands ready to assist the lesser reality during the day when called upon. However, by design, the ego must be worked through while in physical reality and cannot be passed over. We are all on "ego" trips in physical reality.

As I have said, the greater reality functions during the day although most are not now fully aware of its operations. The greater reality manipulates non-physical events during the day to duplicate, as far as it is possible, the picture of reality held by the lesser reality. For example, if a person sees life in general as good, then the greater reality will create situations in which this view is upheld. I say this now because I do not want the reader to get the impression that his greater reality is something that functions without his control. This is not the case. I will point out later in this chapter how you may prove to your own satisfaction that you do have control over what your greater reality does for you in dreams to affect your awake reality.

Briefly, to review what I have pointed out, your pivotal ideas determine what your attitudes are about any given subject. Establishing a direct channel from your answer bank will be based upon the acceptance of this one pivotal idea. Expecting an answer, ask yourself the question. Pivotal ideas may be changed. Your lesser reality deals with physical reality. Your greater reality deals with non-physical reality. Within your greater reality is found an important information center. In order to learn what a part of you already knows will take time. Developmental processes in physical reality are gradual. A certain amount of preparation for the lesser reality is needed to accept information directly from your greater reality.

The first step in learning about the "unknown" is to alter your awake and sleep patterns. Long awake and sleep patterns cause the lesser reality to harden and be unwilling to accept information directly from your information center located in your greater reality. Using our imaginary egg analogy again, when you boil an egg the yolk and the white of the egg become hard and inflexible. Positions become fixed and rigid. Long awake and sleep patterns act on our lesser and greater realities the way boiling water does on the egg. Positions become fixed and rigid.

By altering your long awake pattern with a short nap right after dinner, you begin to regain the natural flexibility of your lesser reality. This nap right after dinner will also give the body time to rest and recharge mental batteries.

This nap at dinner time will cause you to require less sleep at night, thereby indirectly causing you to break up your long sleep period at night. Five or six hours of sleep at night will be sufficient for most individuals to rest the body. If no such new arrangement is made, you can effectively block a direct channel from your answer bank because the lesser reality will not have the needed flexibility to accept data you are looking for.

I happened to discover this at school when I first began to accept direct learning or quiet thoughts from my answer bank and experienced vivid telepathic communications. While I do credit my intense desire to learn this information for bringing forth this data, I was also helped by changing my sleep patterns. At the time, I worked at the university as a night time security guard. I was awake all night and slept for about five and-a-half hours in the morning.

As you are learning to break up excessively long awake and sleep patterns, you may wish to try and prove to your satisfaction that your dreams do influence your awake state. (This is not a step in the process of developing new talents.) For example, by giving yourself the dream direction just before you go to sleep "I direct that I have a dream in which I awaken fully refreshed for tomorrow's activities," you should find that you awaken fully refreshed and ready for the day. However, even without this specific dream direction, the general health of the body is promoted

156

by breaking up excessively long awake and sleep patterns.

To help myself become more efficient at work, I use this direction: "I direct that I have a dream in which I am most efficient at work." When I feel that I am working too hard, I give myself the opposite direction just before I go to sleep. I found the connections were easiest to make when I gave, on alternate nights, opposite dream directions. After I made the connection between my awake activities and dream directions, I made it a nightly practice to program specific dreams, which I rarely recalled, to accomplish certain activities the next day.

You may not at first be able to notice a difference in your behavior the next day but there will be a difference if you accept the idea that your dreams do affect your awake activities.

After you have adjusted your sleep patterns you will be ready to undertake the second step in learning about the "unknown." The second step is to give yourself a specific dream direction. The dream direction is "I direct that I have a dream in which I become aware of any blockages that prevent me from learning direct answers to my personal questions." The purpose of this dream direction is to call upon the greater reality to provide you with any information on blockages in a manner best suited to your personality. If you decide to recall the specific dream, then you will remember the dream because this way is best suited to your personality. But it is not necessary that you recall, remember, or interpret the dream.

Blockages are ideas you now hold which prevent you from learning directly from your information center replies to your personal inquiries. I would like to illustrate what blockages are and how they affect your behavior by the use of an analogy. This time I am going to use an imaginary road. The road surface represents channels in a brain.

Car and truck traffic represent information. Under ideal situations, traffic on this road is free-flowing in both directions, from the greater reality to the lesser reality and vice versa.

However, on our imaginary road that represents channels in your brain going from the greater reality to the lesser reality, no direct traffic or information passes. The cars or information take a detour or use a circuitous route going from the greater reality to the lesser reality. In most instances the reasons for the circuitous route are because of normal blockages or ideas held on the other side of the road, going from the lesser reality to the greater reality. This is because the greater reality is dependent upon the lesser reality for the way physical reality is viewed. If the lesser reality says that data cannot or does not directly originate from inner sources, then this is the view that will be duplicated by the greater reality and no information passes directly. You have a roadblock created by lesser reality because of the ideas it accepts and not the other way around, as you might originally suppose. It may be easier for you to understand the point I am trying to make in the analogy if you draw a diagram illustrating what I have said.

Once you understand the analogy and the point I am making, you will be better able to understand that your thoughts do create your experiences. To make my point clearer, if you hold to the idea that "I can't create a direct channel to my personal answer bank," then you won't be able to do so, because of this idea you now hold. This view you hold in the lesser reality or ego will cause the greater reality to create this situation. If you change this pivotal idea that "I do have a direct channel to my answer bank," then this channel will be created by your greater reality.

In developing new talents, a person must deal successfully with negative ideas or blockages and then accept new pivotal ideas that will cause the talent to be created.

A direct channel of information from your data bank exists only as a potential source of information until the blockage is removed. You will be able to handle the removal of most normal blockages using the procedures I am going to present. Unless you have already developed the ability to experience having your questions answered directly, I am going to assume that a normal blockage exists which can be corrected easily.

In view of what I have just said about blockages, and after you have adjusted your excessively long awake and sleep patterns, I am going to ask that you give yourself this specific dream direction, three times to make sure your mental intention is fixed, just before you go to sleep: "I direct that I have a dream in which I become aware of any blockages that prevent me from learning answers to my personal questions directly from my personal answer bank."

Now, while you are resting your body, your greater reality will be at work presenting the information to your lesser reality or ego. Again it is not necessary that you be able to recall or interpret the specific dream. It is necessary to give the direction.

You may use your own choice of words. It is your mental intention that will cause the greater reality to fashion a way in which the data will be understood by your awake self.

The third step in this process is for you to write on a piece of paper the ideas that you feel create a blockage in a friend of yours from being able to learn answers directly from his or her personal answer bank. This step should follow on the day after you have given yourself the specific dream suggestion in step two, or as soon as practical afterwards.

There may be several ideas which come immediately to mind. I am asking that you let your imagination go for a moment in this step.

Write down any ideas about your friend's blockages that come to mind, no matter how trivial or serious. If you have never thought about your friend in this way, give it some thought. There is no rush; take your time in this step, or in any other step, for that matter.

For example, you may have written down that your friend does not want to believe a personal answer bank exists. You may have said your friend has a know-it-all attitude. You may have to put down your friend is too smart or not smart enough to open a direct channel to his answer bank. Or that he wouldn't want to learn of a personal answer bank because he would then have to accept your list of reasons for blockages. Turn the paper over and put it to one side for a while.

The fourth step in this process is to write down on a piece of paper the ideas that you feel create blockages and prevent you from learning answers directly from your personal answer bank.

You are looking for any negative ideas or contrary opinions that keep you from believing that you can learn answers directly from your own answer bank. There may be one idea or several ideas that come to mind; write them down. If you must give it some thought, do so. Any negative ideas that you have are not deep down in the psyche; they are just unobserved.

For example, you may say: you are too close-minded, you haven't got the time, the process would take too much effort, you aren't interested, or you are unwilling to accept responsibility for your own life.

It is necessary to write down those negative ideas on a piece of paper to objectify your ideas. Objectify means to step outside yourself and see you as you really are. You want to be able to look at these ideas from the outside as the artist looks at his canvas. Like the artist, you want to be able to make changes in the picture you paint with different ideas. I say this now because some readers will consider themselves too smart to write down these negative ideas and then not understand why this process did not work for them.

Step five in this process is to identify, using both lists, the main or pivotal ideas.

What you have done in considering your friend's ideas is to project your personality upon his. You may not be immediately willing to recognize this in the list you made up about your friend or to accept that these negative ideas are your negative ideas. But consider your personality honestly for a moment in view of what you have said about your friend. Most people will find they have unwittingly said something about themselves in what they have written. If you have projected your personality, add this list of reasons to your negative ideas.

Now consider both lists and identify the pivotal or main negative ideas. There usually is only one pivotal idea and the other ideas are subordinate. The pivotal is the idea that you feel is most important. For example, I have decided that the most important or pivotal idea in my illustrations of negative ideas was "an unwillingness to accept complete responsibility for his life." It seems the other ideas are subordinate to this one.

Step six in this process is to deal successfully with the negative pivotal idea and accept a new positive pivotal idea.

We deal successfully with negative ideas when they are no longer a part of our personality, and when we accept new positive pivotal ideas to replace the idea we once held. To achieve this new facet of our personality, we use our effective wishful thinking technique. This technique, which has been discussed before, is a formalization and recognition of what you might do to change your personality. To illustrate how this technique might be used by a person under stress condition to quickly change his personality, let us say you are in a room with a small group of people. A sarcastic acquaintance you have always done your best to avoid makes a loud embarrassing comment about you. Everyone in the room turns his head towards your direction. You want to crawl under the door and away from that person and the group. You are hurt. It does not matter whether what was said was true or untrue; you feel embarrassed.

Instinctively you may deny out loud what was said about you. Immediately you imagine yourself as being the opposite person and give reasons to support this view.

If the comment is true, the embarrassment prompts within you the strong wish or desire to be the opposite person. The embarrassment makes you mad enough to act on this new idea of yourself to prove to others and yourself that you are not the person you once were or that your sarcastic friend imagined.

From the moment of your embarrassment you found reasons to support yourself, even momentarily, that you were not the person spoken about and were, in fact, a new person.

When you boil down our effective wishful thinking technique as illustrated by the analogy to change unwelcome aspects of our personality to more welcome traits, you can arrive at certain guidelines about changing your personality. The first guideline is to deny as no longer being a part of you that negative pivotal idea which causes you to act in the way you do. The second is to imagine yourself as being that positive pivotal idea that will cause you to act in a different way. The strength of the desire for personality change or action will determine the length of time required to actualize this new idea in physical reality.

When I follow the guidelines of our effective wishful thinking technique to change unwelcome personality traits or a normal blockage, I arrive at the following sentences that fix my mental intention, and upon acceptance, bring about the change of personality: "I direct that my unwillingness to accept responsibility for my own life was a part of my personality and experience. Now in this new instance I fully accept responsibility for my life."

By concentrating or dwelling on these sentences for a period of time daily, a person will change, using the example of our normal blockage, his personality in this area. I decided the opposite idea of fully accepting responsibility for his life was the positive pivotal idea needed by this person to properly prepare him for his new role and for quiet thought material.

In arriving at your own sentences, I would recommend that you deal only with the main or pivotal negative idea. Other supporting ideas will change as a direct result of you dealing successfully with the main negative idea. Your own best judgment about what new positive pivotal idea may be needed will prepare you, psychologically speaking, to deal with answers from your personal answer bank.

Few individuals should feel the necessity to deal

with more than one main negative pivotal idea. However, if this is the situation, deal with this other negative idea by adding another mental intention to your statements and supplying another positive pivotal idea which you feel will be beneficial. Some persons who feel personality is fixed or that they are too old to change will also have to deal with these negative pivotal ideas in the same manner.

Many individuals will find that they can successfully change their personality traits, using the effective wishful thinking technique, within a month. Some who have to deal with more than one main negative idea may take longer. There will be instances when an individual is not able to remove normal blockages after trying this method. In these instances, you may be doing so for the overall good of your personality. For example, by removing the blockage, you might concentrate on developing intuitive rather than intellectual abilities. You, through the workings of your inner logic system, which closely monitors your unique development, have decided this. You will permit the removal when you are ready. Each of our blueprints for development is different.

Individuals in situations in which other than normal blockages have to be dealt with may wish to avail themselves of competent help whose opinions and techniques they respect.

Persons who are unable to remove blockages are cautioned against hammering away at themselves and trying to make an alternative work for them that is not suited to their personality at this time. Be assured that a strong desire for answers will prompt inner mechanisms to present answers to your questions in a manner suited to your personality.

Once you have taken the necessary steps to identify and remove blockages and also prepared yourself to accept quiet thought material through a positive pivotal idea, you are now ready to undertake the next step of this process or alternative.

Step seven in this process is the creation of the ability to directly learn answers from your information center. This new ability will be based upon the acceptance of the pivotal idea that you have the ability to learn answers directly from your answer bank.

As a result of accepting this one pivotal idea you will create the attitude that you have this ability. Other subordinate ideas will group around this new main idea to form a particular attitude. Once this attitude is created, you may begin to ask any personal question you wish answered. But until this attitude is created you should not begin to ask personal questions.

The lesser reality, because it deals in physical reality, likes to think that external sources are the only means of information. You have accepted those ideas which trained it to behave in this manner. The lesser reality likes to think it can do the job all by itself. We are going to instruct our lesser reality that it has the ability to look toward both inner-sense or quiet thought information and external-sense or intellectual information which you now use. Using our imaginary egg analogy, the white of the egg will return to an earlier infancy state of being able to look both ways before it becames hard-boiled.

We create this new direct channel of inner communication with ourselves by actualizing an innate potential. Using our road analogy again, once the roadblocks have been removed on the other side of the road going from the lesser reality to the greater reality, we can now build anew the road or channel from the greater reality to the lesser reality. Until the roadway surface is totally completed, no traffic will be invited to pass through premature personal questions. The surface will be completed only when you have the firm attitude or conviction that you already have the ability to directly learn answers to questions from your answer bank.

The formation of this channel or roadway is achieved through the acceptance of a new pivotal idea. The new pivotal idea you want is "I have the ability to learn answers directly from my personal answer bank in the form of quiet thoughts." We apply our effective wishful thinking technique to achieve this new talent. We are simultaneously going to successfully deal with any possible remaining negative ideas and also prevent any new negative ideas from creeping in until the roadway is completed. This may be achieved by giving ourselves a particular direction that states clearly our mental intention. For example, "I direct that I set aside all contrary views I hold about being able to obtain answers directly from my personal answer bank. All these negative ideas were a part of my personality and experience."

It is strongly recommended in formulating your exercise, which you intend to dwell upon for a short time daily to make it a part of your belief system, that you do not direct yourself to answer all personal questions using direct quiet thoughts from your answer bank. If you do give yourself a direction of this sort you may develop too much of an introspective personality. Our goal here is to develop more of an introspective personality and to find answers using inner sources, but not an all-introspective personality.

The mental exercise I am providing may be used by you as a guideline in arriving at your own personal exercise which you feel comfortable in using. Any exercise that you decide upon may be altered and changed if you decide a modification is necessary.

The suggested exercise to achieve the new ability to learn answers directly from your answer bank is as follows: "I direct that I set aside all contrary views I hold about being able to obtain answers directly from my personal answer bank. All these negative ideas were a part of my personality and experience. Now in this new instance I suggest that I have the ability to learn answers directly from my personal answer bank in the form of quiet thoughts during either an awake or sleep state."

As far as it is possible, the greater reality will duplicate this new view held by the lesser reality. The time required to bring this about will vary from individual to individual because we are all unique.

Step eight is to provide reasons to support yourself that you are already the person you want to be. You do this by visualizing yourself as already having benefited by this new talent and by doing a small physical act daily to convince yourself the new talent is already yours.

For example, if by developing the ability to answer personal questions you hope to solve family or business problems, visualize yourself as already living in a happy home or buying things with the new income you will have. The small physical act may be writing daily notes to a friend telling him about your happy home life or your new success in business.

Step eight may be done in conjunction with or subsequent to the mental exercise you decided to follow in step seven.

Briefly, now, let us review the process thus far. Change excessively long awake and sleep patterns; give specific dream suggestions to become aware of possible blockages; project possible blockages on a friend; list your ideas about possible blockages; identify negative pivotal ideas, deal successfully with negative ideas; accept new pivotal ideas; convince yourself you already have the new talent; visualize yourself as already having benefited by the new talent; and do a physical act daily to confirm for yourself that you already have this new talent.

Up to this point, I have been concerned in my illustration about developing the mental ability to directly answer questions using your own personal answer bank. As I said before, this process may be used to develop both mental and physical talents from telepathy to being a good baseball player. You will, of course, have to adapt this technique to whatever talents you want. For example, let us say you have decided to become a baseball player. In step eight, you will have to make a substitution and playfully visualize yourself as already hitting .350 or making key double plays. This step should be accomplished even before spring training. During the baseball season you will live up to this new image as far as possible.

Step nine is to coddle the ego, or lesser reality, for a time until it becomes used to the new talent or role you have asked it to play. If we do not coddle our sometimes timid egos for a time, we may scare the ego into retreating to its former position.

When you first learned to talk, you made garbled sounds much to the pleasure of your parents. Do not be concerned whether the answers you first receive are right or wrong or even if you are learning replies directly from your personal answer bank. With such doubts, you may scare the lesser reality into returning to its former position of dealing only with external sensory perceptions. If this happens, you might find yourself back at step one. As with most new developing talents, the process is gradual. The lesser reality has been trained to act only in a certain way. Now you are training it to act in a far different way. You are going to be using a part of your brain that may not have been used before. A period of adjustment is necessary.

During this time, I am going to strongly suggest you use questions about your own body language as your starting point. I am not going to say that the replies you learn are unimportant. I am going to suggest that these particular replies will be neutral. I hope you are not going to base a course of action on the basis of what you learn about your body language. This area of interest for most people may serve as a stepping stone for resolving more important matters.

It is specifically recommended that you do not begin with personal questions regarding religion or theology because the answers you obtain may be totally opposite from what you currently accept. For example, you might ask yourself the question, "Do devils or evil spirits tempt me?" and you might have this quiet thought, "No, devils or evil spirits do not exist." This quiet thought is a correct answer. However, if previously you believed otherwise, then you would not be building confidence up in your ability to answer personal questions. An ability and confidence to handle replies completely opposite to what you now accept as being correct comes with practice. After you have practiced sufficiently, I recommend any area of personal interest including theology and religion. But at first I suggest a more neutral starting point.

To begin learning about your neutral body language, write down those questions you want to have answered. I suggest that you take about a week or so and base your questions on your own gestures and movements. It will be a good idea if, during the time you are assembling your questions and for the first two weeks when you actually begin to ask yourself questions, you continue the exercises you decided to follow in steps seven and eight. This should be done at a different time of day than when you ask yourself questions.

The question you ask should be phrased in a simple direct sentence. For example, "Why do I cover my mouth with my fingers before speaking?" Long paragraphs are not to be used.

You will find you are more interested in learning answers to some questions than to others and are drawn to certain categories or types of body language.

For example, you may have sixteen questions on feet and hand gestures, ten questions on clothes and only three questions on the positions of the head and shoulders in speaking. Take whatever questions you want answered and separate them into general categories. The reason for this separation and the two week assembly period is to narrow our focus of attention for a time to a particular area and prepare our egos further to accept inner sense information. It will be a matter of personal choice about which category of questions you will decide to answer, using either the awake or sleep states.

After you have compiled your list of questions and separated them, you are now ready to begin asking your questions. For example, the questions about my hand movements I selected to be answered during a quiet moment of the day are: why do I cover my mouth with my fingers before I speak?; why do I scratch the back of my head?; why do I place my hands on my hips?; and why do I tap my fingers on the table? During a time of day when you are least apt to be disturbed or distracted, pull out your list of questions and begin answering them. Answer one question at a time. After you ask yourself the question, wait for a moment or two for the reply to come if you do not have an immediate idea or explanation. Use your imagination for the ones you are not able to answer right away. Again do not be concerned if you do not get an answer or whether the answer you get is right or wrong, or even if you are getting answers directly from your answer bank. Do not spend more than fifteen minutes answering your questions. After this short period, turn your attention away to something else.

The next day, pick another category of questions or finish the remaining questions from your first category. Once again, pick a quiet moment to answer those questions you have, preferably when you are thoroughly rested and mentally alert to catch these quiet thoughts. Do not exceed the ten or fifteen minute period you have allotted yourself. There should be no strain whatsoever in this exercise. If you get stuck on a question, imagine yourself performing or actually perform the same body movement, as you are doing this, listen for the explanation. Or picture a friend using that particular body language gesture and the reason that he is using the gesture. When you have pictured or imagined the reason for your friend doing it, you will know why you do it. You have in all probability projected your personality upon his. If you are unable to come up with a reason or explanation, you may be blocking this quiet thought because this is not what you want to hear. Put this question aside for now until you have better developed your ability.

Continue with this daily exercise for a period of time. You should be able, during other times of the day, to pick up more questions you want answered for the next day. Or you may decide to put meanings to the gestures you make during this ten or fifteen minute period. Now the replies you get on your body language are valid. The reasons why you do a certain gesture may or may not be shared by other people. Body language, like the symbols you use in your dreams, is a personal matter, subject to individual interpretation. Your interpretation of your own body language is superior to anyone else's interpretation. You may see another person using the same gestures. Remember the reasons that he uses the same gestures you do may be entirely different. A green field in one person's dream may symbolize youth and in another's dream old age or retirement.

Now, the answers you get to your questions in this exercise, if you have done this properly and have not heard or read about these meanings before, are quiet thought or intuitions. You have introduced yourself to what quiet thoughts are and have also learned something about yourself. This is the way I first experienced quiet thoughts. You have also cleverly introduced yourself to an unwritten and unspoken form of communication on a conscious level.

After working with your questions for a short time while you are awake and developing a certain level of confidence in your abilities, you should now be ready to pose questions from the category you saved to be answered while you sleep. These questions should be answered the next day in the form of quiet thoughts that you have already been able to identify.

The technique involved here is very simple. It is a matter of giving yourself a direction just before you go to sleep and before you ask the single question you want answered. Later, and with practice, you may ask multiple questions. The direction serves to tell your greater reality that your ego self is prepared to accept the answer and that you become aware of the answer to the question you pose. For example, "I direct that I have a dream in which I become consciously aware of the answer to this question: 'Why do I wear flashy clothes?'" Repeat this direction and question to yourself to make sure you have fixed your mental intention.

After you have successfully experienced getting replies to your body language questions the next day using your sleep state in the form of quiet thoughts, you may then decide to increase the degree of difficulty in your questions. Later, when you have moved into answering other types of personal questions, remember to keep even the most difficult question you want answered in as simple a form as possible.

It is not necessary that you remember the exact dream in which you provided the lesser reality with the information you seek, or even that you be able to interpret the dream as such. Your direction to yourself that you become consciously aware of the answer causes your awake self to become aware of the answer. You should, of course, pay attention to the quiet thoughts you have the next day so you don't miss the answer. If you don't immediately catch the quiet thought, ask this same question to yourself again at the regular quiet moment period, using those same procedures discussed, to identify the exact reply to this question.

The continued expectation that your questions will be answered directly by your answer bank will ultimately lead you to materialize this experience. The neutral area of interest with which you have begun your series of personal interrogations was purposely selected so you would not harm yourself if the replies were based, for a time, upon your conscious imagination. I have allowed about a month for this channel to become a physical reality by developing and using a section of your brain not actualized before. Some persons will take longer than a month and others a shorter period of time. Because of the differences of chemistries, backgrounds, and persons that we all are, there is no hard and fast rule I can draw that will enable you to tell at first the difference between your conscious imaginative material and genuine answer bank learning. Nor will I be able to tell you, how to tell the difference, once you have established a direct channel to your answer bank, between answer bank material and conscious imaginative material, which may slip in on occasion. This is something that you will have to work out for yourself, although a working knowledge of projections or quiet thoughts verbalized will certainly help you to tell the difference.

By and large, after you have gotten your feet wet, you will be able to tell the difference between conscious imaginative and answer bank material. Getting your feet wet without fear of drowning is what the neutral body language training ground is all about.

My experience in being able to tell the difference is not based upon my quiet thought shorthand I alluded to earlier. For example, when I asked myself what would happen *if* heather was used by the New York organization, I had this quiet thought: "Findings confirmed." Although I knew what both words meant, neither was a part of my everyday vocabulary. It was an agreement, in a sense, I made with myself to use a particular choice of words that would catch my attention and identify the reply as a genuine quiet thought. Your experience, however, may be totally different from my experience. I was also helped by learning to expect replies at certain times.

The timing of these replies was often dictated by when I asked for data bank material. If, for example, I asked a question before I went to sleep expecting a reply, without the direction that I become consciously aware of the material, I usually had a reply when I first awoke early in the morning. If I had asked a question and gave the direction to become consciously aware of the reply, I might wake up in the middle of the sleep period with the answer or certainly become aware of the answer early in the morning when I first awoke. Questions posed during a period set aside for quiet thought learning were almost always answered immediately. Questions posed during times not set aside for quiet thought material could be learned anytime thereafter and I had to be careful not to miss the quiet thought.

When your interest in questions about your body language wanes, you should have developed confidence in your ability to use either an awake or sleep state to directly experience answer bank material. You should have developed an attitude based upon the acceptance of this single pivotal idea: "Expecting an answer, ask yourself the question." Now you are able to ask any personal questions and get direct answers to your questions in the form of quiet thoughts. You should ask personal questions using the same techniques that you have been successful with in getting replies to your body language questions.

When I use the term "personal question," I am referring to things that directly affect you. Questions about what to do about the value of the dollar on foreign markets may be within your sphere of interest, but it probably does not affect you directly and therefore does not qualify as a personal question. If you are directly concerned with international finances, then this would be something that directly affects you.

I will deal with questions falling within your sphere of interest in the last chapter of this book.

If for some reason you run into difficulty after having experienced this new talent and "lose" the ability, you may have to begin with step one again. Do not be discouraged if this happens, and you must use the process again to correct the difficulty. I have had to use this same process more times than I care to count to correct situations. Sometimes I was fortunate and did not have to return to step one. Other times I had to go through the entire process to correct the difficulty.

Those individuals who have tried my alternative about learning what a part of you already knows and who are unable to learn directly from their answer bank through quiet thoughts may wish to try at another time. If you try at a later date and are still not successful, there exists the *real* possibility that this alternative is not suited to your personality. A strong desire for answers to your personal questions will bring forward the information you desire in a manner suited to your personality.

I would like to now illustrate how this same technique may be used to resolve a situation in life that you are not happy with and would like to change. Here we are not concerned with developing new talents or an ability to directly answer questions, but rather with giving you an idea about how this practical process may be adapted by you to solve problems encountered in life.

For example, let us say that you have just been laid off from the company where you work and are unable to find immediate employment. You have made the rounds of the employment agencies and cannot find anything you like. Or assume you are told you do not have marketable skills or are too old. Because you have a family to support, you start to make the rounds of the local companies and still do not find any work. "No one is hiring these days," you are told. Three weeks or three months pass and you are still unable to support your family because you cannot find work. You become convinced there are not any jobs or companies are not hiring you for some personal reason. Panic about supporting yourself and your family starts to set in and you are afraid your landlord is going to evict you.

The picture I have painted is not pretty. Those of you who have been without a job may understand what a difficult situation this is to resolve.

Assuming you have become familiar with the

techniques I have presented for learning about the unknown, you may decide to ask yourself, either in your daily quiet thoughts period or before you go to sleep, how to resolve this situation or where you can find work. Then, by paying close attention to your quiet thoughts, act on any new ideas you have to resolve the situation. If you do not have any quiet thoughts or the quiet thoughts that you do have do not resolve the situation, you may have to look closer to the ideas you hold to correct this situation.

"If new talents may be brought about by acceptance of new pivotal ideas," you think to yourself, "then new situations may also be brought about if I deal successfully with those negative ideas I hold, and if I accept new positive ideas." Based upon the principal that the greater reality will mirror, as far as it is possible, those views held by the lesser reality, you are correct in your analysis.

Using the example described, if you are unable to find a job it's because this is the view held by the lesser reality that has been mirrored by the greater reality. When you convince yourself, in spite of the physical fact that you do not have a job, that you do have a job, then this physical event must be brought about by the greater reality. The greater reality acting on the new impulses received will create a situation in which you have a job, after you have dealt with the negative idea.

You begin dealing with the negative ideas you hold by writing them down and seeing yourself from the outside. When you write down the negative ideas, you see that you believe you are too old, your skills are unmarketable, companies are not hiring, and there are no jobs for you. Once you decide upon the main negative pivotal idea, you can now deal successfully with it and accept a new positive pivotal idea at the same time by applying the effective wishful thinking technique. By applying this technique you come up with, using the example of a situation you want changed, a mental exercise you are going to dwell on for not more than ten minutes daily. In this instance you decide to use these sentences to form a mental intention that the greater reality will now mirror: "I direct that all the ideas I hold in the area of there being no jobs for me were a part of my personality. This situation was a part of my experience. I direct that I have a job and I am gainfully employed."

Because I have learned dreams do influence my awake reality, before I go to sleep I would also direct that "I have a dream in which all the ideas I hold in the area of there being no jobs for me were a part of my personality. This situation was a part of my experience. Now in this new moment I have selected a different experience. I direct that I have a job and am gainfully employed."

Daily, after I had completed the awake exercise and given the dream suggestion, I would turn my attention completely away from the situation I wanted to resolve and to another refreshing area of interest. In situations like this, it is important for the lesser reality to shift its center of attention away from the old situation to the new desired situation. Visualizing yourself being benefited by the new job, making a small physical act to convince yourself you already have a job will bring about the new situation more quickly by the greater reality.

It is important to act upon any projections, to solve this situation, or similar situations, by applying these new techniques successfully.

Chapter Six
TELEPATHY

One of the talents that you may have decided to develop by adopting the same method I suggested you use in learning answers from your answer bank is telepathy. Telepathy is the ability to communicate directly with other life forms. This is one talent most individuals assume a psychic has developed. My development of this skill, like many of my other psychic pursuits, has been for personal enjoyment. If development were troublesome, I doubt whether I would have taken the time necessary to gradually develop this talent. I would like to be able to say that learning to be telepathic or receptive to telepathic messages will be learned in one night or two months, but this may not be the case. Once you have developed your own telepathic capabilities, I hope you will find the experience both rewarding and fun.

Sometimes instances of telepathy can be humorous. I was having lunch one day with a group of friends who were generally aware of my psychic abilities and pursuits. One of the young ladies asked me if I could read minds. I said, "Yes, just as well as you can." She sat back in her chair and thought about what I had said for a moment. Then she said, "Can you tell me what I'm thinking?" I replied, " 'No, I will not read what is on your mind' is the answer to your first question and 'No, I will not go to bed with you' is the answer to your second question."

I do not mean to imply that being able to read minds does not lead to some anxious moments or that it is all fun and games.

One night I was at home when I did experience some anxiety for a short time as a result of being able to read minds. If I had not developed the ability, I would not have had a slight case of the jitters. I was living at home with my parents. Because my mother was away visiting my sister, my father and I were bacheloring it. We shared the duties of cooking and taking care of the house and the dog, Ted. After dinner one evening my father and I went downstairs to watch the early evening news on TV. Ever faithful Ted joined us downstairs, but I doubt he was interested in the news. Ted was my father's beloved companion and constant escort. I considered him the ugliest dog I had ever seen and told him so on any number of occasions.

I turned on the TV and sat down in a large comfortable easy chair. I was then nursing a sprained shoulder back to health which I had injured the year before in a cotton field in Israel. I tried to limit my movements, as much as possible, when the shoulder acted up. So when my father asked me to go down to the store a few blocks away to get him a pack of cigarettes, I declined. My father decided to take the short walk down to the store.

As my father was about to leave, I became aware of a telepathic thought that was an unusually strong transmission because of the emotional intensity it carried. The telepathic message was, "I am going out on the street and kill myself."

I was so stunned by the message, I was immobilized. I didn't know what to do. It happened so quickly, I didn't even have time to tell my father I'd go to the store for him.

I sat there for a moment not wanting to believe the message I had picked up. The intensity of the message was so strong that I picked up the message in spite of the fact that my attention was directed at the news on

TV. "How can I stop what is about to happen?" I thought to myself.

If you can picture yourself for a moment being able to read another person's thoughts, and learning someone is about to kill himself, I am sure you will understand the anxiety I felt. There was no mistaking this message or transmission. It was not a premonition because of the wording, "I am going out in the street and kill myself." It was an announcement.

I realized even before this that a person chooses the time, hour, place and circumstances of his death. But this fact of life and death had never been so fully understood before this moment in time. At the time of this psychic experience, I only regretted I had not said good-bye to my father as he was leaving.

I decided to take my mind off the message and the death experience by taking a hot shower. I was still in the shower upstairs when I heard the front door being opened and closed. My father had returned safely from the store. I was relieved. I was also puzzled about how I ever imagined such a terrible telepathic message. I couldn't figure out where I had gone wrong.

I was drying myself when my father knocked on the bathroom door and asked if I had seen Ted, his pet dog. I told him the last time I saw Ted, he was downstairs in the TV room. My father said he wasn't there. Shortly, I heard the front door opening and I assumed my father was going out to find Ted. Five or ten minutes passed, and I was by this time dressed and making my way downstairs. The front door opened and my father was carrying the body of his friend and constant companion, Ted. My father found his body out in the street where Ted had told me he was going to kill himself.

This story of Ted's death is not strange and may be understood when you realize the control that an animal has over his own life. This true story only hints at another world of the "unknown" which may be learned and understood by readers who develop telepathic abilities.

This is not the first instance I have experienced of direct telepathic communication with an animal. I trust it will also not be the last. Modern man has erected a psychological barrier that keeps him from communicating directly with animals. The barrier is as real as a brick wall, but for those readers who are interested in telepathic communications with animals, the barrier may be removed. Those who do not remove the barriers they construct will find that telepathic communication is not possible with either man or animal.

While genuine cases of man-to-man telepathic communications have been documented, the instances of man-to-animal cases of telepathic communications are less frequent and little understood. Because man is able to vocalize and communicate on similiar levels, men in general find the idea of telepathy with another human easier to accept. This is not the case of man-to-animal communication, because the languages spoken are different. It will be easier for a person to accept the idea of direct communication with animals when he realizes that even before his words are spoken, there is mental communication.

I will give some examples, later in this chapter, of this phenomenon that may help a reader understand that his mental communications are understood even before he speaks. Spoken words are an example of the physical clothes mental communications take. Body language is another. It is not necessary to use words to speak to or be understood by either man or animals because your mental communications are already understood.

Nor is it necessary for you to know the different languages both man and animals use before being able to comprehend what is being said, if you allow telepathic communications to become a part of your conscious awareness.

The greater reality, which deals with non-physical events, quite easily handles the communications from both man and animals. This part of you already understands what another part of you pretends not to understand. The pretending is real, however.

Using the same road analogy that was used to explain how your mind functions from your lesser reality to your greater reality, remember that the blockages existed on the lesser reality side of the road. In much the same way, the roadblocks or psychological barriers that keep a person from experiencing mental telepathy exist on his side of the road. You keep yourself from experiencing telepathic communications both from animals and man. In the lesser reality, or ego, which deals with physical reality, you erect roadblocks. These blocks or barriers may be removed and a new channel in the brain developed to handle either or both animal-to-man or man-to-man conscious awareness of telepathic communications.

When I think about telepathy, I think about additions to a five-room house. The five-room house represents the talents you already have. The additions are the new telepathic talents you want. Once you have cleared the land of negative pivotal ideas, you are ready to build your foundation with new pivotal ideas. The walls of the structure represent those new attitudes you will develop. The furnishings represent the individual ways your greater realities will make these telepathic messages known to you. No one furnishes a room exactly the way another person does. How you will become aware of these telepathic messages varies from person to person. We all have different personalities. Your greater reality that knows you best will present the information to your lesser reality when the lesser reality is properly prepared to accept the data and is convinced it already has telepathic abilities. Remember, telepathic messages will be experienced only after you have convinced yourself you have telepathic abilities.

Each person interested in developing telepathic communications will have to deal successfully with his own negative pivotal ideas he now holds in each separate telepathic area. Once the roadblocks or barriers are removed, he will then have to create the new talent based upon the acceptance of new positive pivotal ideas. By adopting the process that I have already fully discussed in the previous chapter, most individuals will be successful in dealing with negative pivotal ideas and accepting new ideas.

I have several reasons for including in this story of a cancer cure a section on telepathy. The first, however, does not deal with the nature of cancer directly. The first reason is to provide a general framework in which an individual may develop his telepathic abilities between himself and members of his own species. The second is that an individual may become more receptive to animal communications. As a result of being able to communicate directly with animals, it will then be possible for interested individuals to directly learn, from animals, the nature of other natural cancer cures.

As you will recall, it is the contention of the doctor with whom I have been in telepathic communication that animals may be used to find other natural cures for all forms of cancer. I am again quoting the doctor's views as learned by me through a series of quiet thoughts.

ANIMALS WHO HAVE THE DISEASE OR WHO HAVE BEEN INJECTED WITH THE DISEASE SHOULD BE INSTRUCTED THAT YOU WOULD LIKE THEM TO LEAD YOU TO A NATURAL CURE. ANIMALS WILL UNDERSTAND IN THEIR MANNER WHAT YOU WOULD LIKE THEM TO DO. ALLOW

THEM COMPLETE FREEDOM TO SEEK THE CURE THEY ARE ALREADY AWARE OF, OR WILL LEARN AMONG THE NATURAL HERBS AND MINERALS OF THE EARTH. ONE AREA TO START THE RESEARCH IS SALINAS, CALIFORNIA. FOLLOWING THIS ANIMAL'S FOOTSTEPS YOU WILL FIND A CURE FOR CANCER. THE KNOWLEDGE YOU SEEK IS ALREADY AVAILABLE TO US. THIS WAY IS BETTER BECAUSE OF THE SYMBOLIC VALUES THAT WOULD BE LOST WERE WE TO USE ANOTHER WAY. THE DISCOVERY OF A CANCER CURE BY AN ANIMAL WILL SYMBOLICALLY STAND FOR OUR ONENESS WITH THE UNIVERSE AND THE ANIMALS OF THIS WORLD, AND SHOW THE SACREDNESS OF EVEN ONE MOUSE. THIS WILL SERVE TO STOP THE UNNEEDED SLAUGHTER OF THE ANIMALS IN OUR LABS BY MEN WHO HAVE GROWN DEAF TO THEIR CRIES. IT WILL BE THE FOOTSTEPS HEARD AROUND THE WORLD. THE NATURAL CURE RESTS OUTSIDE THE CAGES AND BUILDINGS THAT SERVE TO CONTAIN OUR CONSCIOUS KNOWLEDGE AND RESTRAIN ANIMALS FROM SHOWING US THE WAY. WILD AND DOMESTICATED ANIMALS ARE BOTH EQUIP-PED TO SEEK OUT NATURAL CURES. WILD

ANIMALS WILL PERFORM BETTER BECAUSE INSTINCTIVE BEHAVIORAL PATTERNS HAVE NOT BEEN ALTERED. BEFRIENDING OF WILD ANIMALS WILL HELP TO DEVELOP NECESSARY LEVELS OF COMMUNICATIONS. THE TRAINING OF PERSONS SHOULD PROCEED TO ENABLE THESE PERSONS TO BE RECEPTIVE TO ANIMAL COMMUNICATIONS NOW NOT POSSIBLE. THIS WILL MAKE IT POSSIBLE TO LEARN THE INFORMATION YOU REQUIRE DIRECTLY FROM THE ANIMALS WITHOUT THE NEED FOR TRACKING.

I have proved to my own personal satisfaction that telepathic communication is possible between man and animals. I have not tested the doctor's contention that a diseased animal will lead a person to other natural cures for all types of cancers. Nor have I directly or indirectly asked any animal for information on any natural drug cures for any disease. Those persons who are interested in learning of natural drug cures may, where possible, wish to test the doctor's contention on any disease. It is not necessary for a person to have developed telepathic abilities for the animal to understand that you would like him to lead you to a natural cure. I have proven to myself that animals do understand in *their* manner what you are saying when you talk to them, but you will have to ask them either mentally or verbally. As with any direction or request you make, even of man, keep the requests sincere.

I have been able through just casual observation of animal behavior to learn a great deal from animals. And while my observations have nothing to do with telepathy or cancer treatment, I think it would be interesting to make some mention of them here. In a very special way, animals have helped me form opinions on such diverse human topics as marriage, punishment, self-sufficiency and anger, to mention only a few choice topics. If I become confused as to what to do in a particular situation, I do not hesitate to apply natural animal behavior to help form my beliefs or behavior. Here are some of my observations.

Some animals do form special relationships that are respected by their own kind, similar to our special love relationships formed in a marriage. But these animals would never look to man or other animals to sanction the forming or break-up of such relationships. When the purpose of the relationship has been served, they stop the relationship. Either one or both of the animals may decide to stop the relationship and seek to form another one.

Nowhere in the animal kingdom do you find a system of punishment. Killing of other animals or plants for food is not punishment. Animals recognize that, just as they hunted and killed, it may be they will also be hunted and killed for food. Animals do react spontaneously and aggressively to different situations, but their intent is not to punish. Man may also react aggressively to different situations, but the lack of spontaneity may place the reaction into the field of punishment. I trust animals more than any man who believes in a punishment system of justice. Principles of true justice are acted out by the individual in his own way without the need for written laws or punishment codes.

An animal's system of justice revolves around the principle of self-sufficiency. Undomesticated animals provide for themselves. Their existence justifies their right to exist and they do not feel the need to have to prove themselves to anyone.

Animals do not look down unlovingly at their bodies or consider sexual acts as bad or wrong. Without interference from man, animals will maintain a natural balance between their numbers and the environment's ability to support their existence. Learning to live harmoniously with nature, by man taking steps to limit his numbers in proportion to this earth's ability to support his species, is an important group lesson now being learned by man.

If I have learned nothing else from animals, I have learned to be spontaneous. Animals express emotions like anger when they feel angry. They do not, for overly long periods, bottle up emotion until it explodes in a fury. Once vented and fully experienced, emotions like anger change. Attempts to bottle up emotions may cause a person to injure his physical health by his unexamined psychosomatic cause of disease.

A reader who says that animals are only animals does not realize or appreciate his own animal-hood. Man is different from animals, but these differences do not imply being better.

It is true that animals we are familiar with do not have a highly developed specialized part of the brain that we call intellect. More intelligent creatures than man have roamed this earth. Man is now able to make choices among many different alternatives in this reality. In other physical realities, or with some special individuals in this reality, emphasis is placed upon intuitive rather than intellectual development.

Animals, without this highly specialized part of the ego we call intellect, make more efficient use of instinctive learning and are more likely to react to information picked up by their highly developed inner senses, which is ignored by man. Watch dogs use more than just their physical sense perceptions to warn them of dangers. Most animals react to information picked up by their inner senses about natural occurrences such as floods, storms, and earthquakes long before man becomes aware of these dangers on a conscious level. Our so-called primitive societies made better use of animals to predict these natural occurrences and realized the direct connections between these same natural occurrences and the power of man's thoughts.

Animals do enjoy a sophisticated way of learning and knowing that enables them to understand. Observation of animal behavior is one way of learning how to apply an animal's knowledge to suit our needs and requirements. And while it is always possible for man to turn his attention to the same data available to animals by developing his inner senses to warn himself of natural occurrences such as floods, storms, and earthquakes, the information may also be learned directly from animals. Direct communications with some types of animals through telepathy will make this data available. It may be easier for the general reader to accept the possibility of telepathy with animals when he has observed or experienced telepathy with members of his own species.

Once you have made your observations of how your thoughts are already being telepathically received by an interested listener, you may then be able to observe your thoughts being telepathically received by an equally careful animal listener. With neither animal nor humans will these given techniques always apply. Both animal and humans can totally ignore your telepathic thoughts and not react so you cannot make physical observations. The more interested your listener is in what you have to say, the more apt will be your success in this area.

It may be helpful for those of you who have recognized that dreams affect your awake reality to give yourself this suggestion on the nights before you want to observe telepathy: "I direct that I have a dream in which I am able to physically observe my mental telepathy at work with humans." If you feel you will be more successful with animals, you may give yourself this dream direction example by substituting the word "animals" for humans.

I will give some examples of how you may observe your thoughts being telepathically received by other humans. Your observations may be the same or totally different. I will not give illustrations for you to follow on how your thoughts may be observed in animals. My personal research in this area is not complete enough at this time to present practical illustrations that can easily be duplicated by the reader and not challenged as arising from some other cause other than telepathy. I am more at home dealing with human to human telepathy.

Many careful listeners will find they can detect their thoughts being received by humans with or without the dream direction. Let us say you are talking with a person about a controversial subject. You are both interested in the other person's viewpoint, which you do consider and weigh. Both of you also have strong opinions that you can back up with additional comments. In conversations like these, you usually give your view and the other person answers by giving his opinion. You listen and consider what your opponent has said and try to refute his irrefutable statement. Now, when you get in a conversation of this sort, you may wish to try to see how well your thoughts are being picked up by your opponent. When he is giving his argument verbally, silently tell him your opinion which you might ordinarily say out loud. If things go according to plan, your careful listener will react to your silent viewpoint by giving you his answer. I have had any number of instances when not only was his reply given to my viewpoint, but my silent reply was stated as well. Once you realize you've got a live one on the hook, continue with your silent replies to his verbal arguments.

Essentially, what is happening during telepathic communications is that your respective greater realities are each copying thought waves, internalizing a new duplicated thought wave, interpreting the wave, and then making your lesser reality or ego aware of the thought being transmitted, irrespective of the language spoken or the form of the sender. All this happens in a couple of nanoseconds, quite automatically, without your conscious awareness being disturbed by these mechanical details.

Another method of detecting telepathic communications, which I love to employ during the most casual conversations, is to silently ask questions. When I want to learn something from the person I am speaking with, which might prove embarrassing for that person, and I'm not quite sure if I should ask the question, I'll ask the question silently. The person always has the choice of whether or not to answer. You will be surprised at the number of times your silent questions are answered, even about the most intimate details.

Physical distance from the person is not a factor in telepathic communications. Psychological distance is the ruling factor. However, because of the electromagnetic nature of thought waves, weather conditions may interfere with weak transmissions.

You may be able to prove to yourself that physical distances and objects do not interfere with telepathic communications by asking silent questions during a phone conversation. Here you have a better than average chance of having your silent questions answered than you do in selecting a random time to telepathically ask someone a question and get a response. During a phone conversation you have his attention and interest, which is a very important factor to be considered.

Another technique you may use to prove to yourself, without the need of laboratory equipment, that telepathic communications occur even while you sleep is to direct yourself to communicate an important message during sleep. I stress the word "important" here because you want the person on the receiving end to react to your message without your physical prompting. I might also suggest that you first try this

208

with someone you see daily to confirm a positive result.

The direction you should give yourself is simple: "I suggest that I have a dream in which I tell John Doe this message." Keep the message part of your dream direction as simple as possible.

It will be helpful to change your sleeping arrangements to correlate with the North-South polarity of your electromagnetic thought waves rather than an East-West arrangement. Transmission and reception of telepathic messages will be helped by this change of positions.

Once you have taken the time to carefully notice your thoughts being picked up by either persons or animals, you will be able to accept the reality of telepathic communications. You may then decide to develop an ability to become aware at your ego level of what your greater reality already is aware of. The steps which you may decide to follow to develop the ability to "read" either another person's or an animal's mind have already been discussed in the preceding chapter on new talent development. These steps include changing your awake and sleeping patterns, giving specific dream suggestions, dealing with negative pivotal ideas, accepting positive pivotal ideas, visualizing yourself as already being benefited by the new talent, and making a daily physical act to insure your ego's confidence is maintained in the early stages of development.

The resulting new attitudes will be based upon the new pivotal idea you accept as part of your belief structure. Self-training is the key to development in this area.

If you have decided to embark on a telepathic adventure using animals or man as your starting point, I do have a few specific suggestions to help you along the way. Choose only one of the two areas to begin your development, not both at the same time. When you have fully developed your ability in one of the areas, then move to your second area of interest. Begin your initial testing of telepathy with persons you already have psychic connections with, preferably on a daily basis. Family members are best where open communications are permitted. I am including your household pets as family members. Keep your early attempts to monitor other life-forms' thoughts or mental communications to not more than fifteen minutes daily. Those persons who already find it easy to get along with animals will find success quicker to come by than those who do not benefit from this type of companionship. Keep an open mind and sense of humor about what you are trying.

Telepathy or conscious awareness of other life-forms' thoughts is based upon sound psychological principles. Animals and man are capable of producing thought waves. It is a process that goes on constantly under the direction and command of their respective greater realities which handle non-physical events. Certain sensitive equipment is able to monitor some of these waves that are not seen by the naked eye. The greater realities handle thought wave traffic as easily as a normally-sighted person handles refracted light waves.

Not all animals produce thought waves in a manner similar to the way man's thought waves are produced. Very simple animal life forms use a different thought process. While awareness of the particular thoughts of these very simple animals may be achieved by using the same processes I have discussed to enable a person to become aware of more usual thought patterns and messages, the greater realities mechanical operations may differ. Usually animals and man produce two almost identical sets of thought waves. One set is used for the creature's own uses. One set is released or beamed outward. The greater realities of man or animal duplicate the transmission with their own set of thought waves. This new duplicated thought wave is now internalized. The duplication which happens at the point of intersection is not exact. If the lesser reality, or ego, permits the experience of telepathic thoughts, then the greater reality will take steps to present the information.

If the lesser reality or person does not accept the ideas that telepathic communications are possible, then this will be the experience of the person. If the person is capable of handling telepathic messages, and accepts the reality and possibility of such thoughts, then telepathic messages may become a part of his awake reality. It may happen that a person may be directing his attention elsewhere at the time a telepathic thought is received, and the message may be missed. I became aware of a telepathic message from my father's pet dog, Ted, because of the emotional intensity behind the thought. As you will remember, I was watching TV at the time and not paying any attention to Ted. Ted did understand I was mentally talking with him on other occasions. The time I picked the unsolicited message corresponded to the times I usually talked silently with him in the evenings.

Egos, because of the ideas accepted about the

nature of life, are not always willing to readily and clearly accept these messages. Hence you may find your early efforts in this area garbled. The physical channel in the brain must be cleared of all other traffic to allow relatively unhampered data through to become a part of conscious awareness. Even when the way is cleared, messages will not always be exact because of the imperfect duplication process I mentioned. You will color every message with your personality. Those messages that you are not capable of handling will not become a part of your awake reality. You will be more apt to pick up messages that support views of reality that you already hold. Equally valid opposing views may be denied or ignored by the lesser reality. You will permit the experience of happy thoughts when you are predisposed to happy thoughts. A gloomy person will have the opposite experience.

Before you speak a word, the thought that gave rise to that word is internalized by the person you are speaking with long before the words are heard by his physical senses. It is true the words first spoken still ring throughout creation. Thoughts have a reality all their own. Once a thought is beamed outward, it may be shared by others. Each thought bears the stamp of the sender.

Neither the animal nor man thought waves I have been speaking about are the same as the nerve impulses sent throughout their respective bodies. The external thought waves I have been speaking about are not unlike radio or TV broadcasting waves. Greater realities are capable of both duplicating and handling the data in such a way as to be understood by the lesser reality.

Self-training in the area of telepathy will enable you to handle more and more information capable of being provided by the greater reality. Because the ego cannot be circumvented in awake physical reality, there is a gradual developmental process involved.

Individual egos of man and animal may be selective and ignore transmissions or not even bother to acknowledge ego-understood telepathic transmissions. There must be a willingness to respond to telepathic messages that cannot be forced. This is why the befriending of animals is helpful to develop these necessary levels of communications, for animals to do what you request. The animal will understand, if you are sincere in your request, and may react accordingly.

Persons who hold negative views about another individual's telepathic abilities may find their views upheld, even in situations with a person who has demonstrated telepathic abilities. What is happening is that the genuinely telepathic individual's negative views about himself are being acted out. Were this same person to have his positive views supported by those around him, his telepathic abilities might be better demonstrated. When a person asks me to prove my telepathic abilities by reading his mind, I may react to the negativeness he has already demonstrated by making a request that he be more positive.

Telepathy will not always allow someone to read another's thoughts. Certain thoughts are earmarked private, which will be respected by the receiver who will pretend not to know. The pretending is real.

Those individuals who decide to fully develop their man-to-man telepathic abilities will, I am sure, be able to understand men who speak a language foreign to their conscious knowledge.

I am equally sure that those individuals who embark on the psychic adventure to directly understand animals through telepathy will soon be able to put meanings to the different languages spoken by our animal friends.

Chapter Seven
THE ORIGIN OF AN IDEA

Once you have become familiar with the contents of your own personal answer bank through quiet thoughts and have experienced telepathy with either man or animals, you may wish to try your hand at receiving answers from an external answer bank.

I am going to say from the start, beginners in psychic research and those using the approaches I have mentioned should allow themselves at least two years before attempting to test the validity of material in this chapter. If you jump the gun, you may find my suggested methods do not work because you have not properly prepared your egos by using inner resources to accept answers from an external answer bank. Therefore, no valid information may be learned.

It is strongly suggested you confine your questions

to your sphere of interest. Your familiarity with the subjects you want information about will make it easier for you to handle telepathic communication. My telepathic communication with the doctor was severely hampered because of my lack of biological expertise, particularly when dealing with the effects of the drug heather within the cell. The same knowledge may have been learned by a biologist in one night, but it took several weeks for me to gather the data and make it somewhat intelligible. The ego may not be by-passed in physical reality, and hence the necessity of proper ego preparation.

To correct any ego shortcomings, it may be necessary for you to rely on guidance from your own answer bank. When I first asked the question regarding the movement of freight by sound, I got this reply: "Because you are not convinced of the need to know, there is no answer." To by-pass this shortcoming of my ego, I selected the "needed to know" question relating to a natural drug cure for cancer. Later, however, I learned through a quiet thought that I could learn how to move freight practically by using sound, but I would first have to study thermodynamics or physics for three years to understand the data. You may not have to undertake the same program I would to understand this same data. This information on using sound as a source of energy is still available. Sound was used by the Egyptians to build the pyramids.

Some readers may have to educate further their egos in their field of interest in addition to studying the guidelines I will present in this chapter.

The ways I will present to allow you to establish telepathic contact with a source of answers from an external answer bank must be adapted to suit your personality. If you are not comfortable with my specific exercises, you will have to rely for guidance on your own personal answer bank. You will also have to be extremely patient with yourself, not only in making corrections as you go but also in recognizing that developmental processes of telepathic abilities in physical reality are gradual. One step at a time and one question at a time was my motto.

If you do rush the process and become discouraged and quit because you fail in learning the answer to a question, remember you may have had good results if you had taken your time to do your ego preparation homework. Those who say the method will not work are correct. My method will not work for any person who holds that this method will not work because of this same negative view they now hold. A person must be open-minded to adapt this process to his personality.

If you have already developed a personality that is open to telepathic communications, you may now wish to test for yourself my now-accepted contention that an external answer bank does exist.

I would liken my own contact with this answer bank to a visit to an unseen, unexplored, and uncharted but inhabited island. I have only caught a glimpse of one inhabitant, the doctor, and only a glimmer of what might be learned. Both the glimmer and the glimpse was made possible through telepathic communications. I wrote for myself an unusual but natural ticket. Readers who are interested in making such an exploration will have to essentially write their own ticket.

Part of my purpose in writing this story of a cancer cure was to provide a documentation for the origin of an idea and to also help others create their own access to this island.

What may be learned from an external answer bank?

You may answer this question for yourself directly by shifting your attention to another aspect of the reality in which your past and future events are seen as the present. In this spacious present, you may see what new inventions and concepts have not yet been materialized by man or an old invention or idea disregarded by the present civilization. You may also establish telepathic contact with an individual who can also share this overview and learn the answer to your question from him. Or you may decide to accept the opinion of a person who had directly experienced such a perspective of the spacious present or who is in telepathic contact with an individual who had such a perspective. By selecting one of these processes available, you will be able to learn of past or future inventions and ideas that await discovery by man in this age.

The paucity of material I have presented in this book is indicative that the explorations have only begun, rather than of what this external answer bank contains.

A reader must have more than a passing interest in information from an external answer bank, in most cases, to obtain answers. He must actively take the necessary steps to obtain this information. Your current position or wealth will not get you there. Nor will wealth, your current position, or your present age by themselves keep you from obtaining the data you seek. Your sincere interest or desire will enable you to remove the blocks, however natural or normal. The blockages are psychological in nature and exist within us.

The data you seek may be learned telepathically by your greater reality, and then this learning may be passed on to your lesser reality in a way suited to your personality. It may be that the way best suited to your personality is not in experiencing a direct awareness of telepathic communications, in which case you may lead yourself to a particular external physical source of information although this idea springs from some external non-physical source. Direct awareness of telepathic communications is usually not the way "new" ideas are learned.

Usually data from an external answer bank on "new" concepts or inventions is presented to an individual in a dream state. He may or may not even remember the experience. After the information is learned by the greater reality, the greater reality then selects the means by which the information is to be presented to the individual. Hence, the origin of an idea sometimes stems from sources outside the individual, although he may not consciously be aware of how he learned about the new invention or concept. This learning process is done with the full approval of the greater reality. Tacit approval is given by the lesser reality. The person may learn of this full approval by not limiting himself to seeing only his ego-self and by not blinding himself to another equally valid part of his nature.

I consider the doctor I am in telepathic communication with to be only one source or container of information; there are others. Surely these other personalities or life-forms with different experiences will gladly provide us with more information if they are not already providing men with the benefit of their experience. The entity or personality you may establish contact with will depend upon your interests. I am sure there are artists, musicians, engineers, designers, psychologists, teachers, builders, chemists, and biologists who stand ready to assist us.

You do not necessarily have to become aware of the sender to become aware of "new" ideas. If you find contact with an unseen personality objectionable, you may hide the source from yourself or it may be hidden from your ego-self. When I started to learn data on a cancer cure, I was more intrigued by the communications themselves than in the provider of the data. After I became ego-used to the idea of obtaining answers, I learned who was responsible. I did not have a case of the creeps. I considered telepathic communications like a telephone conversation with an unseen friend. I realize telepathy may seem at first glance to be unusual, but it is a natural occurrence. In some ways, telepathy may be more natural than talking through a phone's plastic part over a maze of copper wires with an unseen friend.

Much of what I have learned through telepathic communications has been included in this book in one form or another. My travelogue for development of this psychic ability has already been presented in this story. I have reduced this travelogue to a series of steps that you may now wish to adapt to your personality requirements to learn the new talent of being able to telepathically learn answers from other entities. As your starting point, I am now recommending you use all the same guidelines or steps contained in a previous chapter, "Learning about the 'Unknown.' "

Development of this new talent should begin only after you have first immunized yourself from all forms of cancer and, for many, only after you have become familiar with the contents of your own personal answer bank and have either directly experienced animal or human telepathy. Experience in both telepathic areas will provide you with a level of experience from an unseen source of data.

Developing this new talent of being able to telepathically learn answers from an external answer bank — the process included in the earlier chapter is as follows: Change overly long awake and sleep patterns; give specific dream suggestions to become aware of blockages; project possible blockages on a friend; consider your own ideas about blockages; identify negative pivotal ideas; substitute one unacceptable pivotal idea with a more acceptable pivotal idea; convince yourself you already have the new talent you want; envision yourself already being where you would like to be as a result of developing the talent; and create some small physical act to confirm this new view of yourself and take steps to build confidence in your new abilities.

You may run into trouble along the way and experience difficulties in adapting this process to this new talent. If you do have difficulty, you will have to rely on the talent you have already developed of being able to learn answers from your personal answer bank to correct the situation. One sure sign of trouble is stress. If you find yourself under any stressful conditions anywhere along the way, stop what you are doing. Essentially, your ego is saying no to what you are doing. When I have found myself under stress, I usually find that I had not properly prepared my ego, and/or I tried a short cut that did not work. In either case, I usually stopped for a couple of months before trying again. If, after a couple of months of being away from the process, you try again and still come up with a stress condition that you are unable to resolve by using your personal answer bank, consider the real possibility that you should not proceed.

Once you have developed the attitude that you have the ability to telepathically receive data directly from an external answer bank, you are then ready to take the next step.

I call this, "The Secret of the Ancients" because of an unusual twist. You must convince yourself that you are already aware of the answer to the question you want answered. This state of mind only sounds impossible to achieve.

Our original egg analogy of how your mind functions will help explain why this step is taken. The white of the egg represented your lesser reality or ego, which deals directly with physical reality. The yellow of the egg represented your greater reality which deals with non-physical reality. The view of physical reality pictured by the ego or lesser reality must be duplicated as far as it is possible by the greater reality. So, when you convince yourself that you already know the answer to a question you want answered, the answer you want must be brought about by the greater reality. The greater reality learns telepathically the answer, if it already does not know the answer to the question posed and if the answer is known somewhere within the system. Your greater reality, which knows no limits and is unlimited in its capacity for learning, arranges to produce the data your lesser reality has been fooled into believing it already knows.

For example, let us say your interest is in learning how to practically move freight by sound. The first thing a person should do is to insure that he remains as objective as possible and deal successfully with any ideas he may already hold about how sound may be used to move freight. These views may be correct, partially correct, or totally incorrect, so they must be dealt with to remain objective. You should objectify by writing them down. Once you have written them down, you may now achieve the necessary state of objectivity by using this statement as a preamble to your mental exercise: "I direct I withhold judgment on all views I hold in the area of moving freight by sound as being views of reality which may or may not be correct."

Next, an individual must deal with the negative pivotal idea he now accepts as a part of his belief system. The negative pivotal idea he now holds is that he does not know the answer. As long as you hold onto this negative pivotal idea, this unwelcome reality will be produced and maintained by your greater reality and may short circuit your other positive efforts. As you can see, thoughts are neither positive nor negative by themselves; both are materialized in physical reality. Your thoughts do create both welcome and unwelcome experiences with equal ease. Mysteries of the universe remain mysteries as long as you maintain this view. This negative pivotal idea of not knowing the answer may be dealt with successfully by giving yourself this direction: "I direct that my unknowing was a part of my personality and experience."

Our egos or lesser realities must then either be prepared to directly accept this new information or alert to other means that the greater reality may use to make us aware of the information sought. Again, it is not necessary or always advisable for an individual to directly experience conscious awareness of telepathic communications, so the greater reality may direct the individual to an external physical source of data. As a result of the contact with this external information source, the person may credit his intellect with finding the answer. The following written mental intention will help reassure your ego that you will work through it and not try to by-pass its function: "All interior channels for information are open and functioning to directly experience telepathic messages, if needed, and I am alert for any possible selection of external source information."

The following statement will prevent conflicts from arising between your old negative pivotal idea and the new pivotal idea you will accept: "There is no stress condition experienced because I do this of my own accord."

This phase of the process is completed by telling ourselves our lesser reality is already aware of the answer. "I direct I am already aware of how to practically move freight by sound." This new positive pivotal idea should now become a part of your belief system.

When you assemble all the statements that reflect your new mental intention to be brought about by both the greater and lesser realities, you arrive at the following: "I direct that I withhold judgment on all views I hold in the area of moving freight by sound, as being views of reality which may or may not be correct. I direct that my unknowing was a part of my personality and experience. All interior channels for information are open and functioning to directly experience telepathic messages, if needed. I am alert for any possible selection of external sources of information. There is no stress condition experienced because I do this of my own accord. I direct I am already aware of how to practically move freight by sound." These directions may be used by you as a guideline in establishing your own plan to become aware of answers in your own sphere of interest. Remember, a strong desire for the data is the key, after you have dealt successfully with any negative ideas you hold about obtaining answers.

By dwelling, for not more than fifteen minutes daily, on the mental direction you have formulated to bring about answers to your questions, it should be your experience that you learn the answer. A reasonable length of time is needed, of course, to bring this about. Your experience in obtaining answers from your own personal answer bank will be a good gauge of how long you should continue this exercise. After a period of time, your greater reality, if everything goes according to plan, should manipulate non-physical events to present this information to your lesser reality. The experience you have gained in dealing with the contents of your personal answer bank will enable you to identify how this information will be presented. It may be experienced in the form of a direct quiet thought, a projection, a telepathic message, or indirectly through some external physical source of information such as another person or book.

Theoretically, you may become aware of an answer overnight by using this method, particularly when the data you require is directly associated with your sphere of interest. Practically speaking, this method will not work for the majority of people the first time because they did not properly prepare their egos. These individuals will have to rely on answers from their own answer banks to clear up the difficulty. Some individuals will score the first time out and no further work will be required.

If you have devoted a reasonable length of time to following the mental directions you have prepared for yourself and have not as yet been successful, give yourself a specific dream suggestion to obtain the data for three successive nights. For example, "I direct I have a dream in which I consciously become aware of how to practically move freight by sound."

Follow through on any new ideas obtained. Your first quiet thoughts, projections, feelings, or telepathic messages may be garbled or fouled up. Continue the exercises until the information becomes clear. Once you have started to learn data, continue asking questions about the subject.

The earliest states of telepathic communications are the most delicate because of your ego, which must get used to a new role it is playing. If your ego feels threatened in any way, it may retreat or sever communications. I relied on close friends to give me support in the early stages of development of my psychic abilities. Some other friends I never told of my psychic adventures because they might not have understood. Until the lines of communications are firmly established, I would advise you to take steps to protect your channels of communication by not sharing your experiences with everyone you meet.

If the methods I have proposed do not work, you will have to rely on your own personal answer bank either to clear up the difficulty or establish your own method for learning about the "unknown." I am sure there are other valid methods available. I am only able to provide you with as much information as I now know about the processes to learn about the "unknown." There is still much that I have to learn.

I have provided you, the reader, with an as up-to-date picture as I can in this book. Any questions or problems any reader has or is concerned with will have to be resolved without any further direct help on the doctor's part or my part. For many practical and personal considerations, I do not accept questions or problems to be solved, regardless of merit, from anyone. I do have private pursuits, challenges, and a life to lead, which I intend to follow. This does not mean I have turned a deaf ear to the genuine needs of my fellow man. Whenever anyone does approach me with either a question or a problem, I do recommend using the same techniques I have presented in this book. The ultimate source of all your answers to all your questions is within. It is up to the individual reader to discover them. He may be better able to discover those answers using the methods I have proposed; if these methods do not work, I have no better words of advice for him to follow.

ORDER INFORMATION:

If you would like to order a copy of **"THE STORY OF A CANCER CURE, BOOK ONE,"** please send your name and address, along with a check or money order payable to The Center for Advanced Psychic Research and Development, Inc. in the amount of $25.95 plus shipping charges.

New York residents please add appropriate sales tax.

Shipping charges:		
	U.S.	$3.75
	Canada	$6.00
	Europe	$10.00
	Australia & Asia	$14.00

Please allow 3 weeks for delivery.

Mail to: **The Center for Advanced Psychic Research and Development, Inc.
Post Office Box 1268
Riverhead, New York 11901**